HEALING HERBAL INFUSIONS

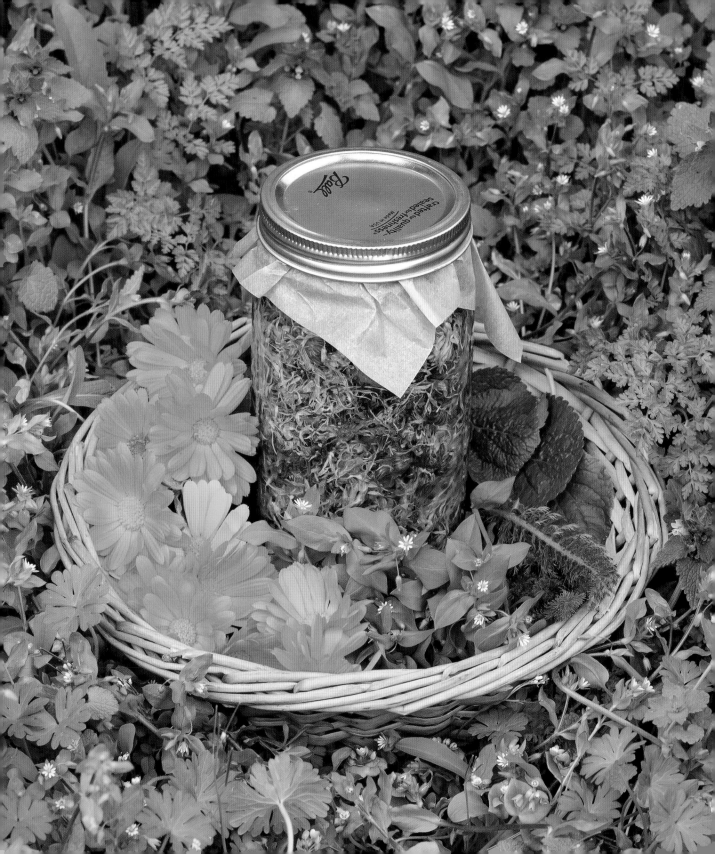

HEALING
HERBAL
INFUSIONS

Simple and Effective Home Remedies
For Colds, Muscle Pain, Upset Stomach,
Stress, Skin Issues and More

COLLEEN CODEKAS

Founder of Grow Forage Cook Ferment

PAGE STREET
PUBLISHING CO.

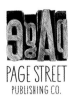

PAGE STREET
PUBLISHING CO.

FOR JOEL AND SAWYER,
MY TWO PARTNERS IN LIFE.

CONTENTS

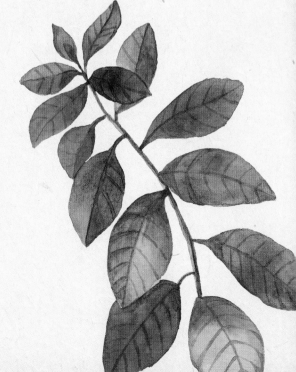

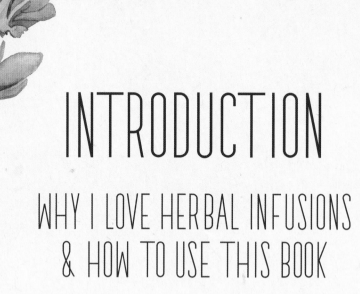

INTRODUCTION

WHY I LOVE HERBAL INFUSIONS & HOW TO USE THIS BOOK

Before I delved into herbalism, much of it seemed difficult or beyond my capabilities. I didn't think that I had the knowledge or skills to make things such as tinctures and salves from scratch. But, when I finally set out to make my first infused oil—after putting it off for way too long—I honestly couldn't believe how easy it was! It was definitely a light-bulb moment for me. I was making herbal medicine!

Putting dried herbs into jars, covering them with oil and then letting them sit for weeks is something that anyone can do. Beyond that, it's merely a matter of choosing the right herbs and the infusing medium that will work best for your particular needs—and this book can help you with that. All that you really need for these recipes are herbs, an infusing liquid and time.

Time. We could all use a little more of it, right? Thankfully, these recipes take very little time to put together. This is the real beauty of herbal infusions and why I love them so much. They do take time to sit and infuse and gather all of their herbal goodness into whatever medium they are infusing into—oil, vinegar, honey, alcohol, water or glycerine. But the best part is that this is unattended time. This is time that the herbs are doing the work for you while you go about your business, waiting patiently for the outcome. What you end up with is an herbal remedy that you can either use as is, like a tincture, tea or infused vinegar, or you can transform it into something else, such as turning an infused oil into a healing salve, body butter or lip balm.

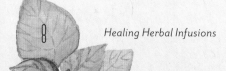

This book is meant to be a guide to help you choose the best herbal remedy for you and your loved ones. I have specially chosen these recipes to cover a wide range of common ailments and issues. Whether you or someone in your family is suffering from a common cold or flu, muscle or body aches, migraines or earaches, upset stomach or heartburn, anxious nerves or insomnia, dry skin or flaky scalp or even has a baby with diaper rash, this book has an herbal treatment for it, plus many more!

The recipes and remedies in this book are all quite simple to make and use herbs that are generally considered to be very safe for the entire family. There are a few exceptions for young children or those who are pregnant or who have specific medical conditions, and they have been noted as such. The formulas that I've included make it easy for someone who is new to herbalism to have confidence in a recipe that is made for a certain ailment. Feel free to adjust the recipes if you'd like, paying attention to the actions of the herbs so that you can find a suitable alternative for your particular needs. The herb profiles at the end of the book (page 191) will help with that. Once you start to understand the basics of herbal infusions, or for those who have some experience making herbal medicine already, you can use the infusion guide at the beginning of the book (page 11) and the herb profiles to come up with your own specific remedies.

When I took that very first infused oil that I made—a mix of calendula, lavender and plantain—and I turned it into a salve, I knew that I was embarking on the beginning of a long herbal journey. It felt right, like what I was meant to be doing. So, during the years, I've expanded on that knowledge, using mostly foraged or homegrown herbs, flowers, roots, berries, bark and leaves. And now I'm so pleased to be sharing all of that knowledge with you in this book. I hope that it will become a part of your herbal journey to natural wellness!

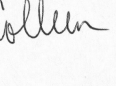

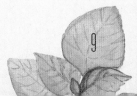

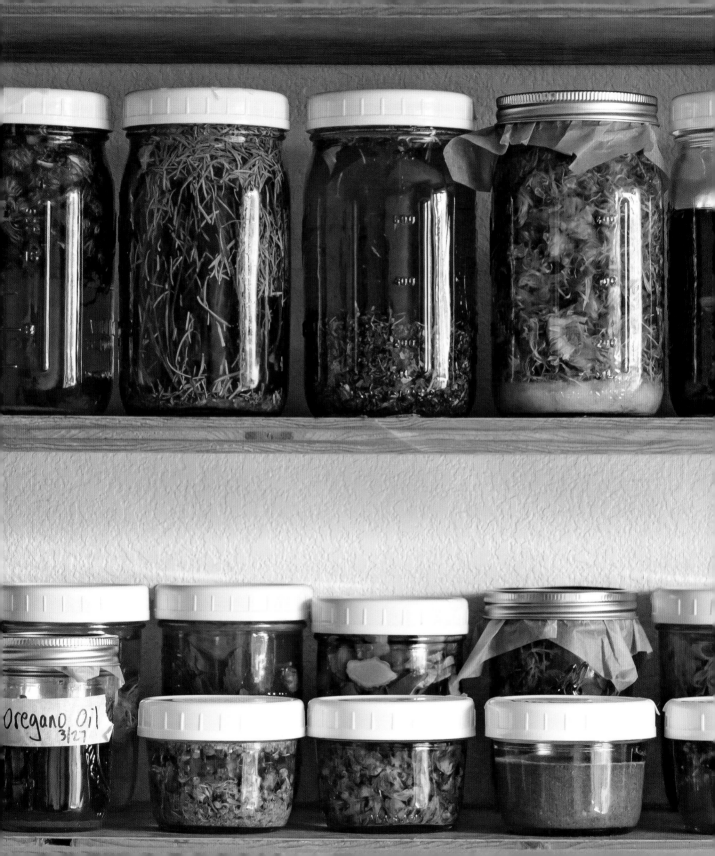

THE BASICS OF HEALING HERBAL INFUSIONS

Before we begin, I have a few tips and tricks for you on how and where to acquire your herbs and flowers. I also explain whether you should use fresh or dried plants—and how to dry them yourself. And I'll give you some basics about the types of infusions that are covered in this book, how to make them and how to use and store them. Refer back to this section whenever you need help or reminders on how to begin or prepare for the recipes to follow. The reference section on page 200 will tell you more about where to purchase some of the ingredients and equipment listed here.

ACQUIRING & PREPARING HERBS & FLOWERS FOR INFUSING

Gathering Your Herbs

Many of the herbs and flowers in this book can be grown in your garden or yard, or they can be wildcrafted (foraged) out in nature. I recommend using both of these methods as much as possible. I always say that the first step in the healing journey is to be out in nature with sunlight on your skin or raindrops on your face, along with getting the blood pumping through our veins by foraging or growing our own medicine.

It is imperative to use a wild plant guidebook or to go with an experienced forager to ensure that you are gathering the right plant. It is also of upmost importance to forage in areas that are free of toxins such as herbicides, pesticides and road runoff. Last, be sure to check where it is legal to collect plants in your area before you go. The following are some herbs used in this book that can be easily wildcrafted in many locations.

- Birch bark (take only from dead or dying trees)
- Burdock root
- Chicory root
- Chickweed
- Dandelion root
- Elderflowers & elderberries
- Hawthorn berries
- Horehound
- Juniper berries
- Lemon balm
- Mullein

- Nettle
- Pine needles
- Plantain
- Red clover
- Rose petals & hips
- Skullcap
- Saint John's wort
- Sunflower
- Uva ursi
- Violet leaf
- White willow bark
- Yarrow

This next group of herbs and flowers is great to have growing in a medicinal herb garden. For the most part, these herbs are easy to grow and require very little maintenance. Some of these herbs are perennial or self-seeding annuals, meaning they come back year after year!

- Arnica (perennial)
- Basil (annual, sometimes self-seeding)
- Calendula (annual, self-seeding)
- Cannabis (annual; make sure it is legal in your area before growing)
- Catnip (perennial)
- Cayenne pepper (annual, sometimes perennial in warmer climates)
- Chamomile (annual, self-seeding)
- Comfrey (perennial)
- Echinacea (perennial)
- Fennel (perennial)

- Feverfew (perennial)
- Garlic (annual)
- Hibiscus (perennial in warmer climates)
- Holy basil (perennial in warmer climates)
- Horehound (perennial)
- Lavender (perennial)
- Lemon balm (perennial)
- Marshmallow root (perennial)
- Onion (annual)
- Oregano (perennial)
- Passionflower (perennial)
- Peppermint (perennial)
- Red raspberry (perennial)
- Rose petals & hips (perennial)
- Rosemary (perennial)
- Sage (perennial)
- Sunflower (annual, self-seeding)
- Thyme (perennial)
- Valerian root (perennial)
- Witch hazel (perennial)
- Yarrow (perennial)

I also list some of my favorite places for purchasing organic dried herbs in the resources section in the back of the book (page 200). This is a great option if it's the wrong time of year for foraging or gardening, for obtaining herbs that are hard to find or do not grow well in your climate or for those who are unable to forage or grow their own.

Purchasing organic dried herbs in the bulk section of your local natural grocery store or food co-op is another good option. This is also a great place to find high-quality, organic fresh plants such as basil, rosemary, sage, thyme, onion and garlic.

Methods for Drying Herbs & Flowers

Many of the recipes in this book call for dried herbs and flowers, so it is a good idea to dry your foraged or harvested plants before using them. Dried plants have a much longer shelf life than fresh, so if you collect elderberries or mullein flowers in the summer and properly dry them, they will be available for use throughout the year.

When your herbal material is fully dry, it will be a bit crispy and dry to the touch. Leaves and flowers should crumble easily. Stems will break when bent, and root pieces will be hard without any give. It is important to make sure that your herbs are totally dry before storing them to prevent mold from forming. Once they are dry, store the herbs in sealed glass jars or paper bags labeled with the plant name and date collected. Keep them in a cool area out of direct sunlight.

Hanging to Dry

This is perhaps the easiest method of drying freshly picked herbs and flowers. Gather them in bunches and tie them with twine. Hang the bunches upside down in a well-ventilated area out of sunlight until they are completely dry to the touch. This method works particularly well with sturdy herbs and flowers that have long stalks or many leaves, such as lavender, yarrow flowers, sunflowers, peppermint and lemon balm.

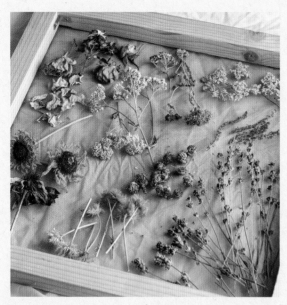

A homemade drying screen is a simple and effective way to dry your foraged or homegrown herbs and flowers.

Drying on a Screen

Use an old window screen, or make your own stackable drying screens with a simple wooden frame and a roll of screening. Spread the herbs out in a single layer on the screen and place in a well-ventilated area out of sunlight until dry. This is a great way to dry individual leaves or flower petals, berries, small flowers or root pieces. It also is the best method for more fragile flowers that tend to fall apart when dried, such as elderflowers.

Using a Dehydrator

A good dehydrator can be helpful if you need dried plant material in a hurry or if you live in a particularly humid area. I have an Excalibur, and there are several other high-quality brands available. Use it on the lowest setting. Check the plants often and remove them as soon as they are completely dry to the touch.

When to Use Fresh Plant Material vs. Dried

Dried herbs and flowers are the safest to use in many infusions as they will greatly reduce the chances of spoilage or rancidity. This is especially true for oil infusions, in which using fresh plant material can even be dangerous due to botulism spores. With the exception of one recipe in which I thought it was important to use the fresh herb (Oregano-Infused Oil with Lemon, page 44), I call for using dried herbs in all of the infused oil recipes in this book. Using fresh herbs in oil infusions is acceptable if you will be using all of the oil within a few weeks.

There are certain types of infusions in which it is perfectly safe to use fresh plant material, and a few in which it is even beneficial because some herbs are more potent when fresh. For infusions that will be stored for a long period of time before use, the general rule is that if it has a high acidity, high alcohol content or high sugar content, then it is safe to use fresh herbs. This is because the acid, alcohol and sugar are all-natural preservatives. This means that alcohol (tinctures and bitters), vinegar, honey and glycerite infusions are all fine to make with fresh plant material.

For tea infusions, either fresh or dried plants will work equally well. Dried herbs are usually more practical for making teas because they are more concentrated, so a smaller volume of herbs is needed. Fresh herbs are nice to use if you have access to them, because they are often more aromatic and sometimes contain more beneficial volatile oils.

If you'd like to use fresh herbs in place of dried, simply use twice as much as what is called for in the recipe.

TYPES OF HERBAL INFUSIONS & HOW TO MAKE THEM

Medicinal Teas, Overnight Infusions & Decoctions

Herbal teas are the simplest and most straightforward of all the infusions, requiring only herbs and water. A medicinal tea uses either fresh or dried herbs steeped in near boiling water, usually for 10 to 20 minutes. The tea is then strained and consumed, usually while still hot.

For a much stronger medicinal tea, try a long or overnight infusion. Put the herbs in a mason jar and add boiling water, then cover and let it infuse for several hours or overnight. Strain out the herbs with a fine-mesh sieve before drinking. These types of infusions are commonly served cold over ice, but they can be gently warmed if a hot tea is desired.

A decoction is made by simmering the plant material in water for 20 to 30 minutes before straining and drinking. This is the best method for extracting the medicinal benefits of harder plant material, such as roots, bark, twigs and seeds. A medicinal syrup is often started by making a strong decoction, then letting it cool before adding honey or another sweetener.

There are some herbs that do better in a cold-water infusion, as some of their healing properties can be lost with heat. Use the same method as the long or overnight infusion described above, but use cold or room temperature water. A few herbs that benefit from a cold infusion are marshmallow root, slippery elm, nettle, lemon balm and comfrey root.

Alcohol & Vinegar Infusions

Infusions using alcohol or vinegar for the liquid medium are popular because they have an almost indefinite shelf life. High-proof spirits (80 to 90 proof is ideal), such as vodka, gin, whiskey, brandy or rum, are highly effective at extracting all of the beneficial compounds from herbs. Tinctures are most often made by infusing medicinal herbs in a high-proof spirit. Digestive bitters (pages 115–116) are made in the same way as a tincture, but use bitter herbs and a neutral spirit such as vodka as the medium, so that the flavor of the herbs comes through.

If you'd rather not use alcohol for tincture making, vinegar is a great alternative (for children I recommend using glycerine; see the next section). Raw apple cider vinegar has many health benefits of its own, and it is preferred for most preparations. It is also a great choice for boosting the immune system (see pages 40 and 43), helping to relieve heartburn (see page 119) and natural hair care (see page 160).

Either fresh or dried plant material can be used to make alcohol or vinegar infusions. Simply put the desired herbs into a jar, then fill it with either alcohol or vinegar. Cover the jar and let it sit in a dark place for 4 to 6 weeks, then strain out the herbs with a fine-mesh sieve before using.

Honey & Glycerite Infusions

Sometimes a sweeter infusion is needed, and raw honey is usually what I reach for in this case. Raw honey is antibacterial, antimicrobial, antifungal and anti-inflammatory, so it has plenty of medicinal benefits on its own. It is a powerful immune system booster (see page 35), and it is effective treatment for minor burns (see page 65), acid reflux (see pages 103 and 119) and sore throats (see page 78).

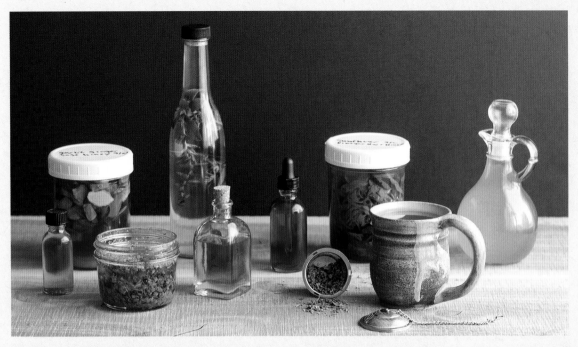

There are many different types of herbal infusions to make for your home apothecary. Shown here from left to right are rose hip serum, fermented garlic and ginger honey, chamomile and calendula infused oil, herbal hair wash, dandelion root digestive bitters, echinacea tincture, vinegar hair rinse, catnip tea and ginger syrup.

Raw honey hasn't been pasteurized, so all of the wild yeast, beneficial enzymes, vitamins and minerals are still intact. The best place to acquire raw honey is from a local beekeeper, or you can also see what your local farmers' market has to offer. If you don't have access to raw honey locally, I suggest purchasing from a natural and organic food distributor such as Azure Standard (see resources, page 200).

If fresh plant material is used in raw honey infusions, the small amount of water present in the plant will "wake up" the natural wild yeast in the honey and it will begin to ferment (see fermented honey recipes on pages 35–36). The end result is a super tasty infusion that is also highly medicinal. If you do not want the honey to ferment, be sure to use dried herbs.

Glycerites are tinctures made with herbs infused in a sweet vegetable-based glycerine syrup (see recipes on pages 186–189). These are typically made for children to make the tincture more palatable, and they are suitable for those wishing to avoid alcohol. Both fresh or dried herbs can be used, but if you are using dried herbs, it is usually advised to also add a bit of water to the mix.

For both honey infusions and glycerites, put the desired herbs into a jar. Fill the jar with either honey or glycerine. Cover the jar and put it in a cool and dark place to infuse for 4 to 6 weeks. Be sure to turn the jar every few days to coat the herbs; this is especially important when using fresh herbs.

Oil Infusions

I must admit, I really love making infused oils. This is actually where my herbal infusion journey began, and I've refined my process significantly along the way. Oil infusions are how many herbal bath and body care products begin, so knowing the process is important if you want to delve into homemade salves, lip balms, lotion bars and body butters.

There are many methods for infusing herbs into oil, and some definitely work better than others. One big problem is that the oil can go rancid or become moldy if done incorrectly. Fortunately, there are ways to avoid that. The main thing to remember is to keep light, heat and water away from your herbal oil.

Cold Infusion

The most effective and safest infusion method is to use dried herbs and to do a slow infusion in a cool and dark place for 4 to 6 weeks. This is the method I use in most of the infused oil recipes in this book.

My main rule of thumb is to use completely dry plant material whenever possible when making herb-infused oils. This is because any moisture that is in the plants can cause spoilage and possibly even cause mold to grow on the surface. There are a few exceptions to this rule, mostly because there are a handful of herbs and flowers that lose their potency when dried, such as dandelion flowers, Saint John's wort flowers, mullein flowers, chickweed and lemon balm. If you'd like to use fresh herbs in these instances, it's best to first slightly wilt the herbs or flowers for a day or so, then use the heat method that I describe next. When using fresh herbs, it's also a good idea to only make what you will use up within a month.

Quick Heat Method

To infuse oils using the heat method, the easiest way is to warm them in a slow cooker on the very lowest setting or by using a double boiler (see tips for making one yourself on page 20). I usually do not prefer this method because heating oils over a certain temperature can degrade them, but in the rare instance where fresh or wilted herbs are being used, this is an acceptable method to use. The heat will cause some of the water content to evaporate while also speeding up the infusion process, so they have less chance of going bad. Keep the oil uncovered to allow evaporation, and heat for 12 to 24 hours. The oil should not be heated over 110°F (43°C), which can sometimes be hard to gauge depending on which method of heating you choose. One trick that I've learned is to heat them in a box-style dehydrator (see resources, page 200) if you happen to have one. It is an awesome appliance that can fit many jars at once and has lower temperature settings, so there is no worry of overheating.

If you need your infused oil sooner than the 4- to 6-week time frame, you can use the heat method with dried herbs as well. The process is the same as described above, but you do not need to leave the oil uncovered while heating, as there is no water content to evaporate. I will often do this when I need the oil sooner than 4 to 6 weeks, then continue to let them sit for a week or two before using. Just remember that the oil will be a little bit more degraded than if you didn't heat the oil, meaning that it will go rancid sooner, but still not as quickly as if it were exposed to water or sunlight.

Solar Heat Method

Another common method for infusing herbs into oil is to place the jar in a sunny window for several weeks. While this can be an effective method for certain oils with higher saturated fat content such as coconut oil, keep in mind that sunlight will degrade many oils considerably and cause them to go rancid much quicker than normal. Because of this, I generally try to avoid using this method.

Helpful Equipment for Making Infusions

Making herbal infusions requires very little equipment, but there are a few items that can make things easier.

Mason jars in different shapes and sizes. You will be making the majority of your infusions in these. I've gathered quite the mason jar collection during the years, and they are used daily in my kitchen. The sizes I reach for most often are half-pint (236 ml), pint (473 ml) and quart (946 ml).

Lids for your mason jars. I recommend not allowing the metal canning jar lids and rings that usually come with mason jars to come in contact with your infusions. This is because the metal can react with the liquid and create an off product. To avoid this, simply put a piece of parchment paper over the jar first, then top with the metal lid and ring. Alternatively, you can purchase plastic lids that fit on mason jars for storage purposes.

Fine-mesh sieves in various sizes. These are important for straining out small herb particles, and it is helpful to have a few different sizes. A piece of cheesecloth placed inside a strainer also works well and will make it easy to squeeze out all of the liquid from the herbs.

A teapot with a strainer, a stainless-steel tea ball or a reusable muslin tea bag. This is essential for making medicinal teas.

Bottles and jars for storing your finished infusions. It's good to have various sizes on hand. Small dropper bottles for tinctures are especially helpful.

A small funnel. This is necessary for transferring the strained infusion into narrow-necked or small bottles.

TIPS FOR MAKING SALVES, BALMS & BUTTERS

Choosing Carrier Oils

When making your herb-infused oils that will be turned into body and skin care products such as salves, balms, lotion bars and butters, it's important to consider what kind of oil to use. In the majority of my recipes, I use a blend of oils to get different benefits that I think will work best for each specific recipe. However, feel free to change it up to your liking, as some people prefer certain oils over others. Here are the oils that I use most:

- *Olive Oil:* This is often the easiest oil to use because it is readily available almost everywhere. Extra-virgin olive oil is preferred. It is vitamin rich, high in antioxidants, hydrating and moisturizing. Olive oil is a great all-purpose oil that can be used in almost any skin care recipe.

- *Coconut Oil:* Solid at room temperature (melts at 76°F or 24°C), this oil is very shelf stable due to the high amount of saturated fat. I prefer to use virgin unrefined coconut oil because the refining process can remove some of its benefits. Unrefined will have a coconut scent, refined will not. It is high in fatty acids, and it is antibacterial, antimicrobial, anti-inflammatory and moisturizing.

- *Sweet Almond Oil:* A popular choice for skin care products because it has a light texture that penetrates easily into the skin and is highly moisturizing. It is gentle and safe for all skin types, and it is a good choice for use on babies, children and those with sensitive skin.

- *Apricot Kernel Oil:* This light and highly emollient oil absorbs readily into the skin. It is rich in essential fatty acids and vitamins A and K, and it is an excellent choice for dry and itchy skin conditions. It is anti-inflammatory, has anti-aging properties and is good for those with sensitive skin.

- *Castor Oil:* A very thick and rich oil that is super moisturizing. It is anti-inflammatory, antimicrobial and good for treating all types of skin conditions. A little goes a long way for adding natural lusciousness and shine to lip balms and salves.

- *Jojoba Oil:* This is not technically an oil but a liquid wax that comes from the jojoba plant. It has a long shelf life. It is excellent for moisturizing and adding shine to hair, and it is used as a treatment for dry scalp. It is most often used in hair and beard care products, but it also promotes healthy skin.

- *Rose Hip Seed Oil:* This light and nongreasy oil is primarily used for its anti-aging properties. It is very hydrating and penetrates the skin on contact, and it can be used undiluted on the face. It is very heat- and light-sensitive, and it should be kept refrigerated and out of direct sunlight.

Waxes & Butters

In order for a salve, balm or lotion bar to set up, some kind of wax needs to be added to the infused oil. I prefer to use high-quality beeswax from a local source (see resources, page 200), as it is naturally hydrating and increases essential moisture in the skin. Blocks of beeswax can be reduced into smaller pieces for easier melting by carefully using a heavy-duty kitchen knife or cleaver to break them into approximately 1-inch (2.5-cm) chunks. Another option for easier measuring and melting is to purchase beeswax pastilles. Alternatives to beeswax include carnauba wax and candelilla wax, but be aware that these are significantly harder than beeswax so less is needed.

Butters don't necessarily need to be added to salves and balms, but they sure make them wonderful! They are also the base for body butters, making them super rich and moisturizing. I recommend using them whenever possible, as they can take your skin care products to the next level. Here are a few of my favorites:

- *Shea Butter:* An intense moisturizer for dry and irritated skin. It is an excellent choice for most skin care products. It is high in essential fatty acids and vitamins A and E. Unrefined shea butter has a strong odor that is hard to mask, so I generally prefer to use a minimally processed refined product.

- *Cocoa Butter:* Super rich and creamy, and high in vitamin E and antioxidants. It is perfect for very dry, cracked and irritated skin. The unrefined version has a strong chocolate-like odor, so keep that in mind when adding it to skin care products.

- *Mango Butter:* Highly moisturizing, skin softening and rich. This is the perfect butter for dry hands. It is also often used on the face due to its anti-aging properties. It is a natural emollient, and it is high in essential fatty acids. Unrefined is preferred, but a minimally processed refined product will also work.

Equipment & Making a Double Boiler

The best part about making salves, balms, lotion bars and butters is that very little equipment is required, and you probably already have most of it in your kitchen. Here is what I recommend having on hand:

- Digital kitchen scale
- Small saucepan
- Glass measuring cup (such as Pyrex) or a pint-size (473-ml) mason jar
- Canning jar ring
- Wooden or bamboo skewer
- Small jars, tins or lip balm tubes
- Molds for making lotion bars
- Hand mixer for making body butters

Because the beeswax and butters can be difficult to completely remove from cookware, I like to have one glass measuring cup that is used only for salve and balm making. You could also use a mason jar for this purpose, but it's harder to pour the hot liquid out because it lacks a spout.

To make a double boiler, put 2 to 3 inches (5 to 7 cm) of water into the saucepan and bring it to a low simmer. Place a canning jar ring on the bottom of the pot, then set the glass measuring cup or mason jar containing the strained infused oil onto the ring. Use the smallest saucepan that you have so that there is no room for the glass measuring cup or mason jar to accidentally tip over. A wooden or bamboo skewer is handy for stirring the melting beeswax and butters and good for mixing in any essential oils you may be using.

HOW TO USE & STORE YOUR INFUSIONS

Using Your Infusions

For the most part, using your infusions is pretty straightforward. In each recipe I include instructions for how much and how often to use them. Here are some general guidelines to get you started:

Medicinal teas are consumed soon after making, either hot or cold, sometimes with a little honey or other sweetener to make them more palatable if desired. Decoctions can also be ingested right away, but are often turned into syrups instead. Medicinal syrups can be taken one spoonful at a time, whether taken straight or diluted into water or tea.

Tinctures are very potent, so only a few drops at a time are needed. They are generally stored in a dropper bottle for this purpose, and they can either be taken straight or diluted with water or tea if desired. Digestive bitters are also very strong, and they are often diluted with sparkling water or used in an aperitif or digestif cocktail (see pages 115–116). Vinegar infusions are acidic and have a strong flavor, so only about 1 to 2 tablespoons (15 to 30 ml) are taken at a time. They can either be taken straight or mixed with water and/or honey.

Honey infusions have a great benefit in that they taste great! Take a spoonful or two at a time, either straight or stirred into tea or water. Children under the age of 1 (as on page 23) should not ingest honey because of the slight chance of the honey containing botulism spores.

Glycerites can be taken in the same manner as tinctures, and they are a good alternative for children or those who wish to avoid the alcohol in traditional tinctures.

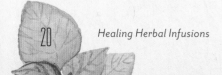

Healing Herbal Infusions

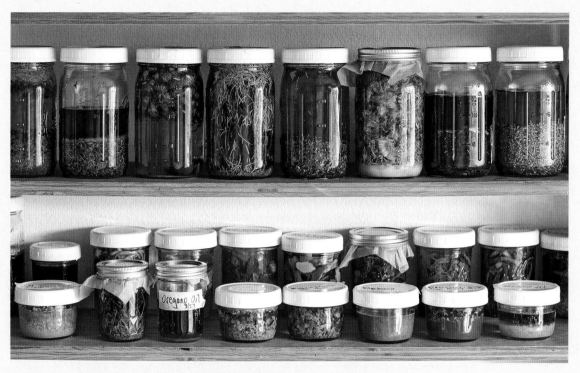

It is important to properly label and store your herbal infusions for increased shelf life.

Infused oils are most often used topically by rubbing directly onto the affected area or made into topical salves, balms and butters. This is especially the case with the recipes in this book. Herb-infused oils can also be used internally depending on the herb and which oil you choose, such as Oregano-Infused Oil with Lemon (page 44). Beyond herbal medicine, some infused oils have wonderful culinary uses.

It's worth noting that use of more than one infusion at a time is generally acceptable, depending on the specific remedy. For example, drinking the Super Immunity Infusion Tea (page 27) along with taking some Fermented Garlic, Ginger & Sage in Honey (page 35) would be very beneficial during times of illness. Adding in a bit of one of the immune-boosting tinctures would also probably be fine, but be careful about the overlap in herbs between the recipes so that you aren't taking too much of one herb. Most of the recipes in this book use herbs that are safe even in larger amounts, so that shouldn't be an issue for the most part, but it is something to be aware of.

Labeling, Storing & Shelf Life

When making herbal infusions, it is very important to label them with a name and the date made. If you're anything like me, you'll soon have several jars (or more!) of various herbs infusing in various mediums, and it is important to know what each one is and when they started infusing. Masking tape and a felt-tip pen work great for this purpose.

It is fine to wait to strain your infusions until you are ready to use them, even if it's after the infusing time period listed in the recipe. (The exception is fresh herbs in oil; those need to be strained and used in a timely manner.) They will only get more potent over time. Store your strained herbal infusions in a cool place out of direct sunlight—a dark pantry or kitchen cabinet is perfect. Amber jars and bottles can be helpful for storing light-sensitive infusions.

Shelf life will vary greatly between each infusion depending on the type of liquid medium and if dried or fresh herbs are used. With infused oils there will be variation based on the type of oil used, as some are more shelf stable than others. In every case, if the infusion looks or smells off, or if it has mold or anything else questionable growing on the surface or within the infusion itself, it's time to compost it.

Infused oils that are made with dried herbs will last for 6 to 12 months or even a bit longer if stored properly. If they are made with fresh herbs, they will only last for 1 to 2 months maximum.

Alcohol infusions such as tinctures and bitters will last almost indefinitely, at least 5 years and probably longer. Glycerites are good for 3 to 5 years, and both vinegar and honey infusions are good for 1 to 2 years.

Medicinal teas are generally consumed soon after making, but if you are making a long or overnight infused tea, you can strain and store it in the refrigerator for several days.

Syrups need to be refrigerated, and they will last 2 to 4 weeks in the fridge. After that they may begin to ferment, which isn't harmful, but may or may not be desired. If you'd like to increase the shelf life of a syrup, it can be frozen in baggies or ice cube trays and then thawed as needed before use.

SAFETY CONSIDERATIONS & DOSING FOR CHILDREN

A Few Notes on Safety

While all the herbs and recipes presented in this book are very safe to use, and I believe that herbal medicine can benefit everyone immensely, there are a few safety considerations that should be noted.

Store all infusions and finished products well out of reach of small children and pets.

Pregnant and nursing women should always consult their doctor, midwife or a trained herbalist before consuming any herbal preparations.

People with serious medical conditions or autoimmune disorders should consult their doctor, naturopath or a trained herbalist before consuming any herbal preparations.

If the herbal preparation doesn't seem to be working, or if the condition becomes more serious, please consult your doctor, naturopath or a trained herbalist.

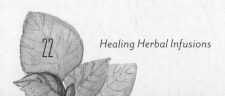

I recommend doing a patch test before using any herbal preparation, especially when they are to be used on babies and children, to make sure there aren't any allergies or irritation caused by a specific herb or ingredient. To do this, rub a small amount on the back of the hand or on the inner arm and wait to see if there is any reaction before using. This can be done with salves, balms, body butters, lotion bars and herbal teas.

How to Dose Properly for Children

While I have several recipes that are formulated especially for babies and children (see Infusions to Support Mother & Child on page 167), many of the recipes in this book are safe to use for little ones. I have noted if the recipe is generally considered safe for children, and if so, which ages. I recommend talking with the child's pediatrician, naturopath or a trained herbalist before giving any herbal preparations to children.

For recipes that are to be used internally, here are some general dosage guidelines for children:

- *Under Age 1:* If the adult dosage is 1 cup (240 ml), the child dosage is ½ to 1 teaspoon (3 to 5 ml). I only have one recipe in this book that I recommend using internally for a baby under the age of 1, Children's Calming Tea (page 185). Nursing mothers have the added benefit of taking the herbal preparation themselves (as long as it is safe to do so) and passing on the protection to their infant.

- *1 to 2 Years:* If the adult dosage is 1 cup (240 ml), the child dosage is 1 to 2 teaspoons (5 to 10 ml). If the adult dosage is 1 tablespoon (15 ml), the child dosage is 5 to 8 drops.

- *3 to 7 Years:* If the adult dosage is 1 cup (240 ml), the child dosage is 2 teaspoons to 2 tablespoons (10 to 30 ml). If the adult dosage is 1 tablespoon (15 ml), the child dosage is 8 to 15 drops.

- *8 to 12 Years:* If the adult dosage is 1 cup (240 ml), the child dosage is 2 to 4 tablespoons (30 to 60 ml). If the adult dosage is 1 tablespoon (15 ml), the child dosage is 15 to 30 drops.

- *13 to 18 Years:* This age group can usually take a full adult dosage, mostly depending on the weight of the child. Those on the younger and smaller end should take one-half to three-quarters of an adult dose.

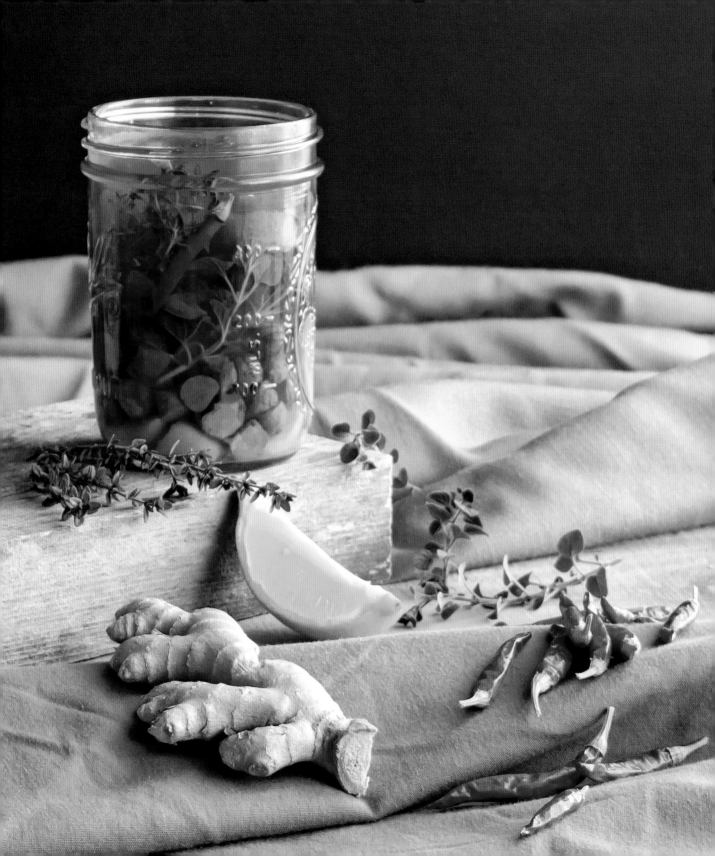

INFUSIONS TO BOOST YOUR IMMUNITY

Our immune system can be a delicate thing, but there are ways of naturally supporting it with herbs. This is especially important during the fall and winter months when viruses tend to go around. Thankfully, there are many herbs, berries, flowers and roots that help to boost our immune system. And, if we do happen to catch something, they also help to provide some relief. Many of these herbs are ones that you may already have growing out in your garden. Beyond their everyday uses in the kitchen, sage, thyme, oregano and rosemary all have powerful medicinal benefits. Others, such as elderberries and rose hips, are easily wildcrafted in most areas. The following recipes for tinctures, teas and other herbal infusions help keep your immune system healthy and keep you feeling well.

25

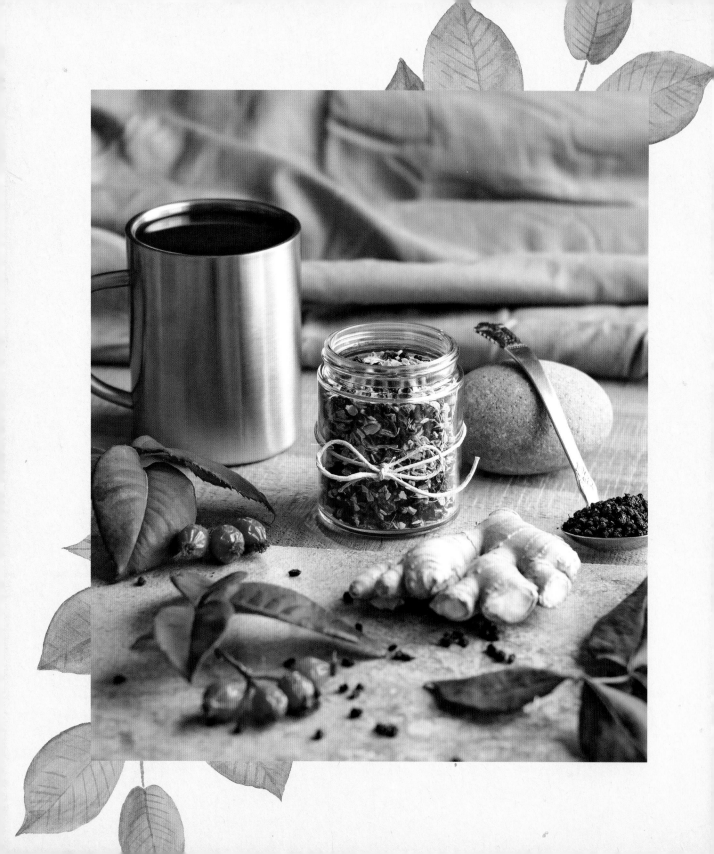

SUPER IMMUNITY INFUSION TEA

When you feel a sickness coming on, sometimes a hot cup of tea is the only thing that sounds good. Choose this super immune-boosting tea to help fight off the bug and to protect you from future ones! I like to use dried herbs in this tea blend so that I can make up a larger batch to always have on hand when I need it. Simply use equal amounts of each dried herb, mix well and store in a glass jar covered with a lid. Use 2 tablespoons per 1 cup (240 ml) of water whenever you need that extra boost to your immune system.

Yield: 2 cups (480 ml)

Ingredients
2 cups (480 ml) water
1 tbsp (6 g) dried elderberries
1 tbsp (8 g) dried rose hips
1 tbsp (6 g) dried echinacea root
1 tbsp (5 g) dried ginger

Instructions
Bring the water to a boil and pour over the dried herbs. Let the infusion steep for 10 to 15 minutes, then strain out the herbs before drinking. For a stronger tea, follow the directions on page 15 for a long or overnight infusion.

Drink 1 to 2 cups (240 to 480 ml) twice per day at the first sign of a cold or flu, or sip throughout the day during an ailment to help shorten the duration.

This tea is safe for children ages 2 and older. Please follow the dosage guidelines on page 23.

Tip: Give the gift of super immunity! Put this beautiful tea blend in a mason jar. Wrap some ribbon or twine around it and add a tag with instructions for use.

VITAMIN C TEA

It has become common knowledge that vitamin C is beneficial for the immune system. Instead of taking a supplement or drinking sugary and acidic orange juice, sip on this hot herbal tea that is naturally high in vitamin C. Rose hips are one of the highest natural sources of vitamin C, and hibiscus flowers have a good amount as well. This tea is a beautiful ruby-red color that can brighten up any dark mood! Pregnant women should avoid using hibiscus.

Yield: 2 cups (480 ml)

Ingredients
2 cups (480 ml) water
1 tbsp (8 g) dried rose hips
2 tbsp (6 g) dried hibiscus flowers
1 tsp (2 g) dried orange peel
1 tsp (2 g) cinnamon chips or ½ cinnamon stick broken into pieces

---

Instructions
Bring the water to a boil and pour over the dried herbs. Let the infusion steep for 10 to 15 minutes, then strain out the herbs before drinking. For a stronger tea, follow the directions on page 15 for a long or overnight infusion. This tea can be consumed hot or iced.

Drink 1 to 2 cups (240 to 480 ml) per day during cold and flu season to keep your immunity up, or sip 2 cups (480 ml) throughout the day during an ailment to help shorten the duration.

This tea is safe for children ages 2 and older. Please follow the dosage guidelines on page 23.

Tip: As an added side effect, hibiscus flowers are also great for lowering blood pressure.

Healing Herbal Infusions

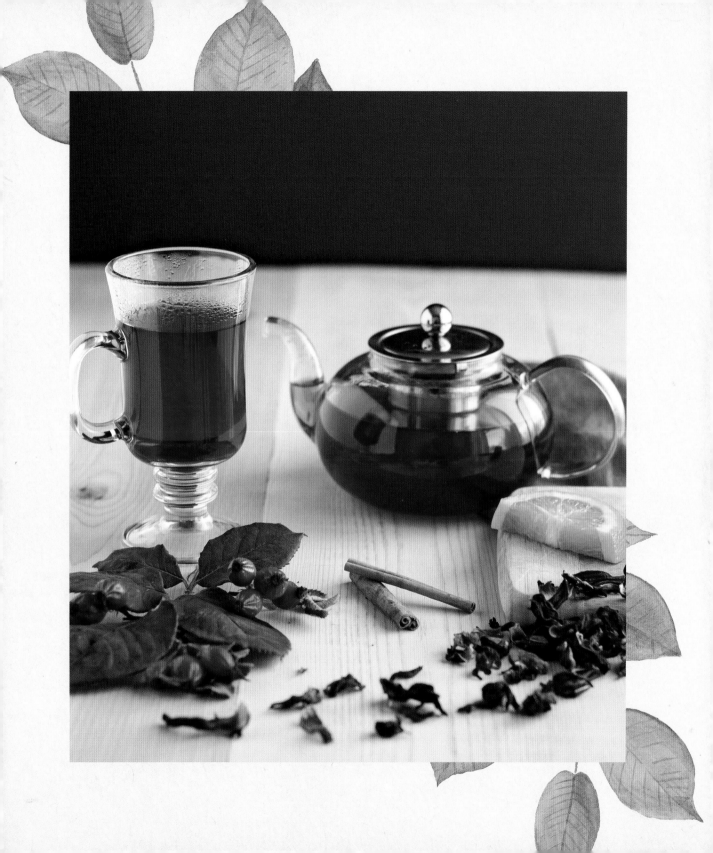

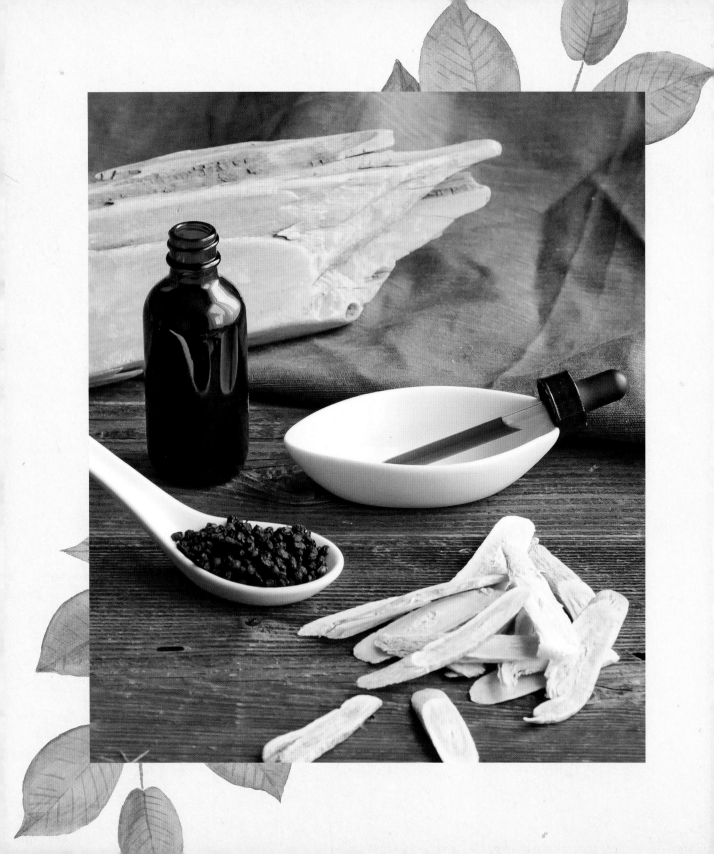

ELDERBERRY & ASTRAGALUS TINCTURE

Both elderberry and astragalus are immune-boosting powerhouses that are commonly used in tinctures. Elderberries are one of my favorite edible and medicinal plants to forage for in the late summer and early fall, which is perfect timing for cold and flu season. If you are using foraged elderberries, one trick for removing the tiny berries from the stems is to freeze the whole cluster first, then they will pop right off! Astragalus root comes to us from Traditional Chinese Medicine, bringing with it a gentle yet effective immune-strengthening response that will help keep you feeling well all winter long.

Yield: about 1½ cups (360 ml)

Ingredients
¼ cup (30 g) dried elderberries

½ cup (30 g) dried astragalus root slices

1½ cups (360 ml) neutral spirits, such as vodka

Instructions
Combine the elderberries, astragalus and spirits in a pint-size (473-ml) jar. Cover the jar with a lid and shake to mix well. Put the jar in a cool and dark place to infuse for 4 to 6 weeks. Strain out the herbs using a fine-mesh sieve. Store the tincture in small bottles with droppers for easy use.

Take 1 teaspoon (5 ml) 2 to 3 times per day at the first sign of a cold or flu for the most benefit. It can be taken straight or mixed into water or tea if you prefer.

For children and those wishing to avoid alcohol, use Elderberry & Echinacea Glycerite for Colds & Flus (page 186), or you can make this same tincture with vegetable glycerine instead of the neutral spirits.

Tip: Astragalus is a safe herb that can be given to the entire family. Some people even like to include it as an ingredient when making nourishing broths!

ECHINACEA ROOT & FLOWER TINCTURE

Almost everyone these days has heard of echinacea, as it has become a rather popular herbal remedy. Echinacea is excellent for boosting the immune system, and it has been proven to shorten the duration of colds and flus. It's also a gorgeous flower to grow in your garden that serves double duty: beauty in your yard and wellness in your home. This tincture is simple to make, and it uses both the root and the flower, making it even more beneficial!

Yield: about 1½ cups (360 ml)

Ingredients
½ cup (40 g) dried echinacea root
½ cup (20 g) dried whole echinacea flowers and/or leaves
1½ cups (360 ml) neutral spirits, such as vodka

Instructions
Combine the echinacea root, flowers and spirits in a pint-size (473-ml) jar. Cover the jar with a lid and shake to mix well. Put the jar in a cool and dark place to infuse for 4 to 6 weeks. When ready to use, strain out the herbs using a fine-mesh sieve. Store the tincture in small bottles with droppers for easy use.

Take 1 teaspoon (5 ml) 2 to 3 times per day at the first sign of a cold or flu for the most benefit. It can be taken straight or mixed into water or tea if you prefer.

For children and those wishing to avoid alcohol, use Elderberry & Echinacea Glycerite for Colds & Flus (page 186), or you can make this same tincture with vegetable glycerine instead of the neutral spirits.

Tip: It's okay if you don't have the echinacea flowers or leaves to add to this recipe. The root is very medicinal on its own and is easy to locate in most places that carry dried herbs.

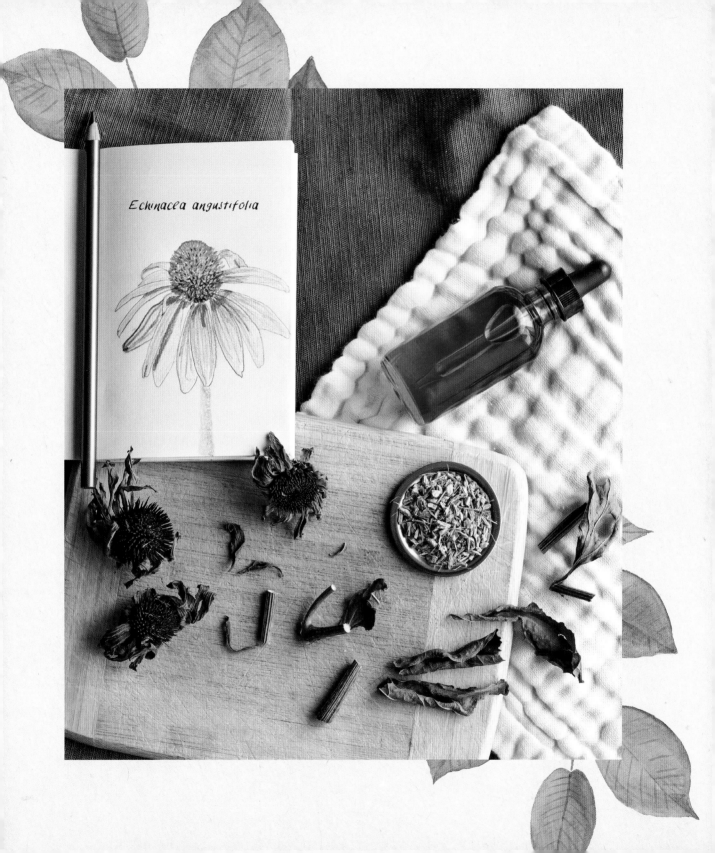

Echinacea angustifolia

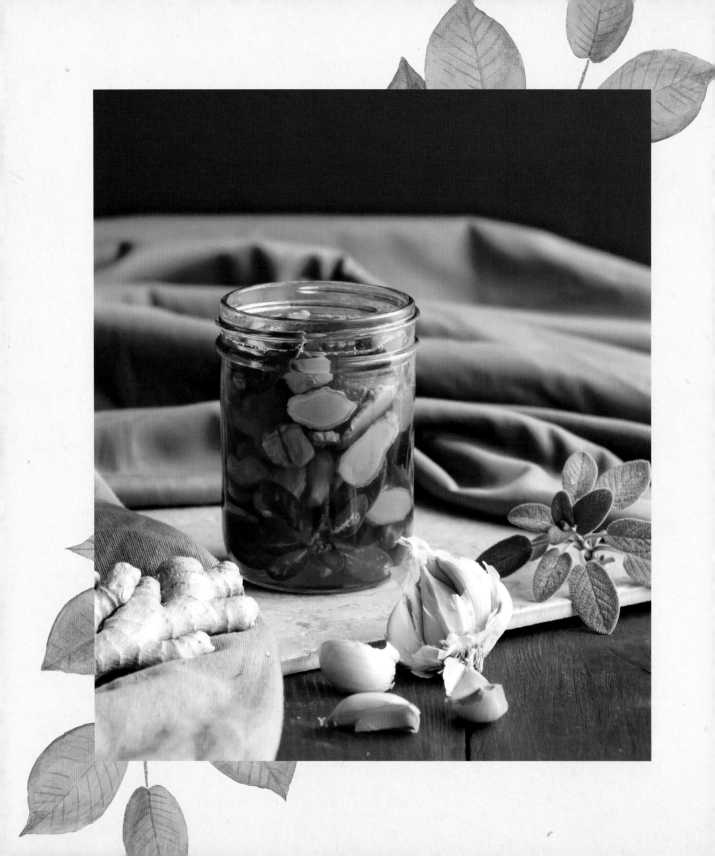

FERMENTED GARLIC, GINGER & SAGE IN HONEY

Fermenting fresh herbs in honey is a tasty way to really boost your immunity. Plus it's fun to make! Raw honey is full of wild yeast and will readily ferment when even a small amount of moisture is added. The water content in garlic is enough to get the process going, and fermented honey garlic is the most basic version. I like to add in some different immune-boosting herbs with the garlic, such as fresh ginger and sage, to make it even more beneficial. Sage is especially good for sore throats and coughs. The honey will get runnier as it ferments, and it will last for a full season or even longer. While this sounds like a strong concoction, the flavor of the garlic and ginger mellows considerably after fermentation, giving you all the benefits of these herbs in a delicious way.

Yield: about 2 cups (480 ml)

Ingredients
2 heads (50 g) garlic, cloves separated and peeled
½ cup (50 g) sliced fresh ginger
2 small bunches (10 g) fresh sage leaves
1¼ cups (300 ml) raw honey

Instructions
Combine the garlic, ginger, sage leaves and honey in a pint-size (473-ml) jar. Cover the jar with a lid and invert it several times to coat all of the herbs in honey. They will probably float and that's normal. Loosen the lid a bit to allow gasses to escape and put the jar in a cool, dark place to ferment. Tighten the lid and turn the jar daily for a week or two to coat everything with honey, then loosen the lid again after turning. In a few days you will start to see some bubbles forming in the jar and the honey will be runny in texture. It will be fully fermented in about a month, but can be consumed at any time during the process.

Take 1 tablespoon (15 ml) of honey, or even one whole garlic clove or ginger slice, whenever you feel a sickness coming on, up to 3 times daily. It can also be taken once or twice daily throughout cold and flu season as a preventative measure and to help boost your overall immunity.

This fermented honey is safe for children ages 2 and older. Please follow the dosage guidelines on page 23.

Tip: Swap out the sage for any fresh herb that you might have in your garden. Rosemary, thyme, oregano and mint will all work well, and they are all beneficial to the immune system.

FERMENTED RED ONION & THYME IN HONEY

This recipe is along the same lines as the Fermented Garlic, Ginger & Sage Honey on the previous page, but this time we're using red onions and thyme. While garlic and ginger are well known for their immune-boosting benefits, not many people know about the benefits of onions! They are high in antioxidants and vitamin C, plus many other compounds that are good for the health. Thyme is one of the most powerful herbs for immunity, and there's a good chance that you already have it growing in your herb garden. Feel free to use any other fresh culinary herb that you have on hand instead, as most of them also have medicinal properties.

Yield: about 2 cups (480 ml)

Ingredients
1 cup (130 g) red onion slices
½ cup (4 g) loosely packed fresh thyme sprigs
1¼ cups (300 ml) raw honey

Instructions
Combine the onion, thyme and honey in a pint-size (473-ml) jar. Cover the jar with a lid and invert it several times to coat the onion slices and thyme in honey. They will probably float and that's normal. Loosen the lid a bit to allow gasses to escape and put the jar in a cool, dark place to ferment. Tighten the lid and turn the jar daily for a week or two to coat everything with honey, then loosen the lid again after turning. In a few days you will start to see some bubbles forming in the jar and the honey will be runny in texture. It will be fully fermented in about a month, but can be consumed at any time during the process.

Take 1 tablespoon (15 ml) of honey, or even a few slices of onion, whenever you feel a sickness coming on, up to 3 times daily. It can also be taken once or twice daily throughout cold and flu season as a preventative measure and to help boost your overall immunity.

This fermented honey is safe for children ages 2 and older. Please follow the dosage guidelines on page 23.

Tip: This also makes a wonderful tasting marinade or glaze for meats or vegetables!

Healing Herbal Infusions

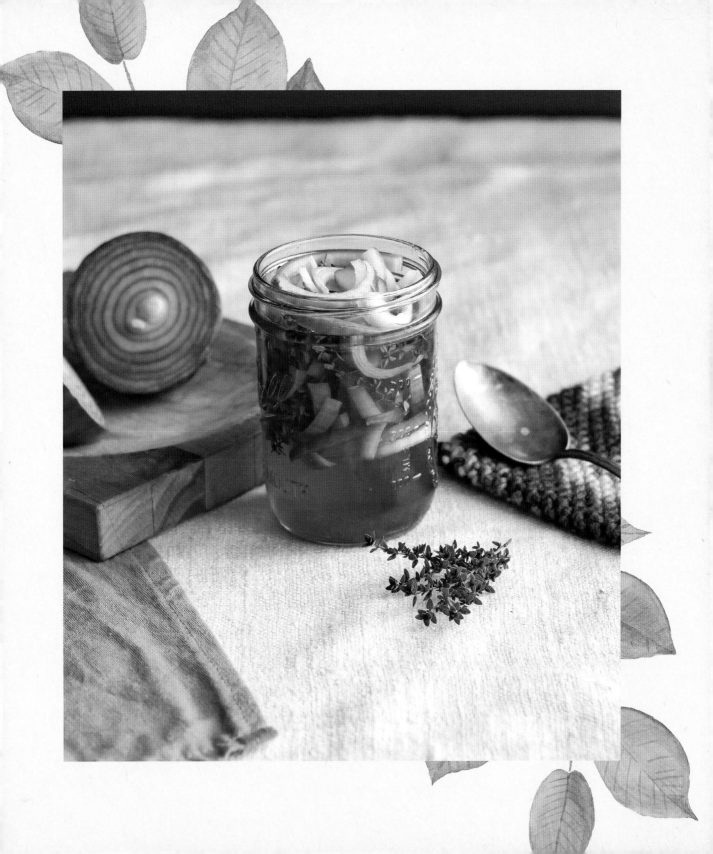

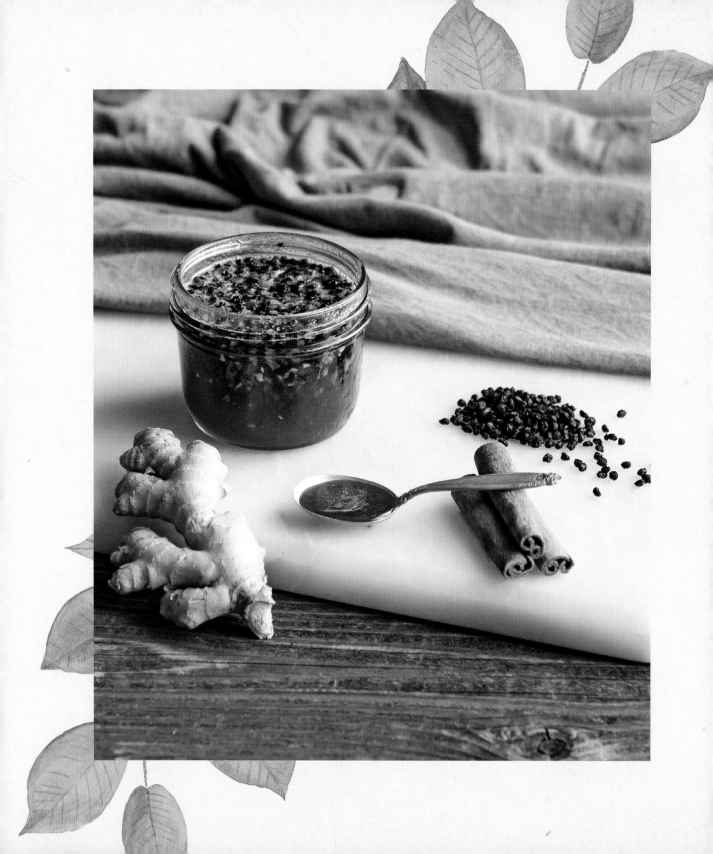

ELDERBERRY, GINGER & CINNAMON HONEY

Infusing honey with dried herbs is a great way to get their benefits in a highly palatable way. Elderberries are one of my favorite immune-boosting herbs, and they are usually easy to forage for in the late summer or early fall. I always make sure to gather enough to dry to have on hand for the winter. Ginger and cinnamon increase the flavor of this honey, while providing even more immune-boosting support. Stir a spoonful of the strained honey into tea, drizzle it over fruit or yogurt or simply eat it as is.

Yield: about ¾ cup (180 ml)

Ingredients
2 tbsp (12 g) dried elderberries

1 tbsp (5 g) dried ginger pieces

2 tsp (5 g) dried cinnamon chips or 1 cinnamon stick broken into pieces

¾ cup (180 ml) raw honey

Instructions
Combine the elderberries, ginger, cinnamon and honey in a half-pint (236-ml) jar. Stir it well so that all of the herbs are suspended in the honey. Cover the jar with a lid and put it in a cool, dark place to infuse for 4 to 6 weeks or longer, stirring or inverting the jar once every few days or whenever you happen to think about it. Strain the herbs from the honey with a strainer when ready to use.

Take 1 tablespoon (15 ml) whenever you feel a sickness coming on, up to 3 times daily. It can also be taken once or twice daily throughout cold and flu season as a preventative measure and to help boost your overall immunity. It can be taken straight, but is also nice when stirred into tea.

This infused honey is safe for children ages 2 and older. Please follow the dosage guidelines on page 23.

Tip: If you use fresh elderberries and ginger instead of dried, the water content in the herbs will create a fermented honey as in the previous two recipes.

FRESH KITCHEN HERB OXYMEL

An oxymel is a mixture of honey and vinegar that is most often infused with herbs and used as medicine. Both raw honey and raw apple cider vinegar are beneficial to the immune system on their own, and even more so when they are combined with healing herbs. I find a ratio of half honey to half vinegar to be perfect—a little sweet, a little sour and goes down easy. In this oxymel recipe, I call for any fresh herbs that you might have growing out in your herb garden. Most kitchen herbs are also medicinal and helpful for the immune system, so they serve two purposes!

Yield: about 1½ cups (360 ml)

Ingredients
1 cup (12 g) loosely packed fresh garden herbs, such as rosemary, thyme, sage, basil, oregano and mint (I use mostly whole leaves and sprigs)
¾ cup (180 ml) raw apple cider vinegar
¾ cup (180 ml) raw honey

Instructions
Combine the fresh herbs, vinegar and honey in a pint-size (473-ml) jar. Cover the jar with a lid, and shake well to thoroughly combine the honey and vinegar. Put the jar in a cool, dark place to infuse for 4 to 6 weeks. Strain out the herbs with a strainer when ready to use.

Take 1 tablespoon (15 ml) whenever you feel a sickness coming on, up to 3 times daily. It can also be taken once or twice daily throughout cold and flu season as a preventative measure and to help boost your overall immunity. It can be taken straight or stirred into water.

This oxymel is safe for children ages 2 and older. Please follow the dosage guidelines on page 23.

Tip: This oxymel also makes a great marinade for meat and vegetables, or combine with some olive oil and you have an instant herbal salad dressing!

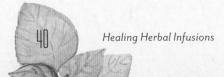

Healing Herbal Infusions

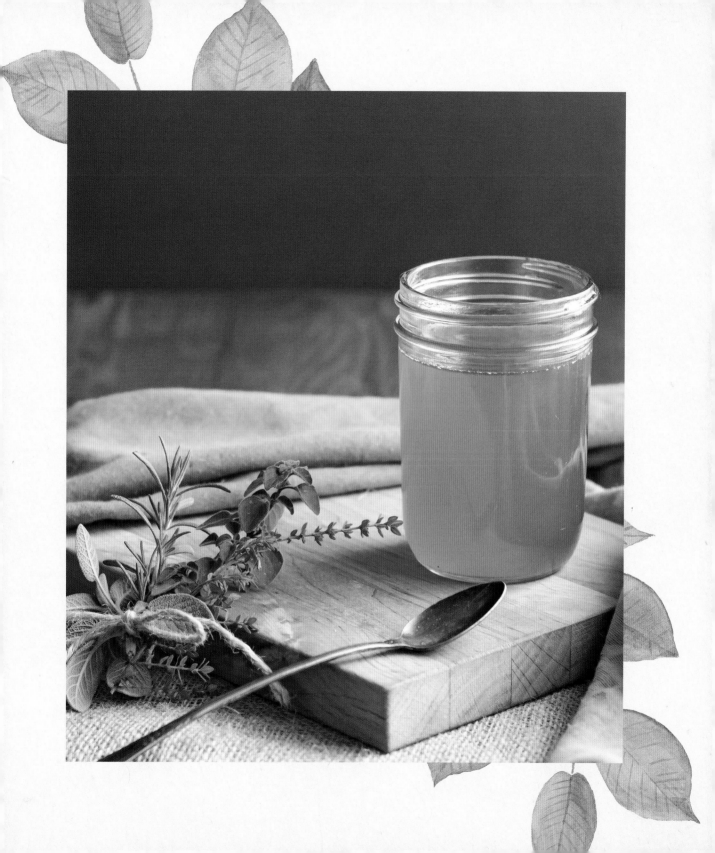

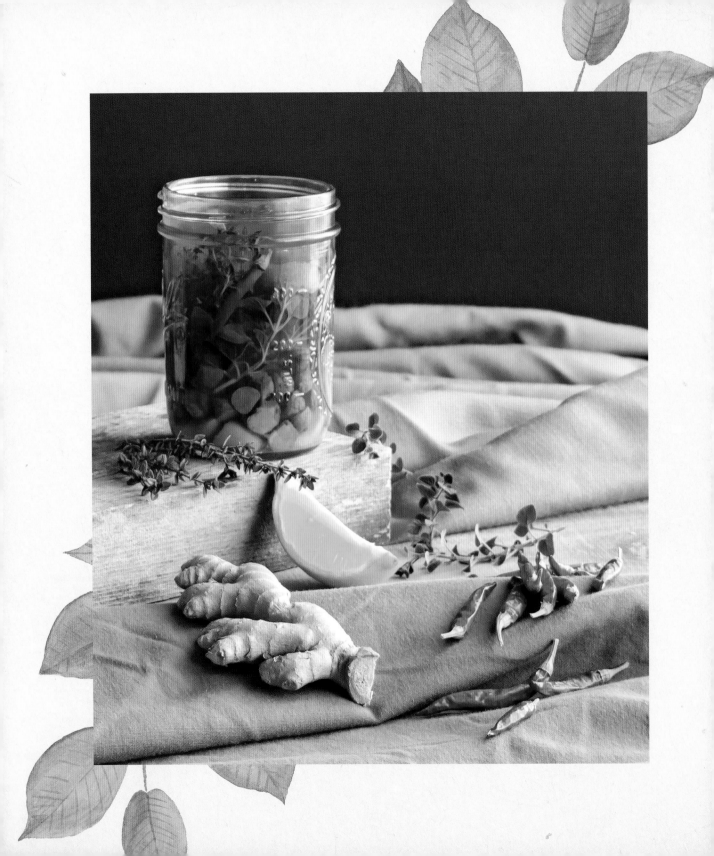

IMMUNE-BOOSTING VINEGAR INFUSION (HOT OR NOT)

Often called "fiery cider" or something similar, an infusion of immune-boosting herbs and hot peppers in apple cider vinegar has become popular in recent years—and for good reason. This is a potent elixir that will put a fire in your belly and keep you feeling healthy all winter long. One question I often get is if the hot peppers are necessary, and the answer is no. While spicy peppers do benefit the immune system, many people can't tolerate them and would prefer to leave them out. This recipe is beneficial to the immune system with or without the hot peppers, depending on your preference. If you do decide to use hot peppers, you can choose something on the less spicy side such as pepperoncini or jalapeño, or go for something super spicy such as habañero or Thai hot. Other options include cayenne, serrano, anaheim and tabasco.

Yield: about 1½ cups (360 ml)

Ingredients

6 cloves (21 g) garlic

¼ cup (28 g) sliced fresh ginger

¼ cup (28 g) sliced fresh turmeric root

Small handful (3 g) fresh oregano sprigs

Small handful (3 g) fresh thyme sprigs

Zest and juice of 1 lemon

1–2 fresh hot peppers, such as jalapeño, cayenne or habañero, sliced (optional)

1½ cups (360 ml) raw apple cider vinegar

1–3 tbsp (15–45 ml) raw honey (optional)

Instructions

Combine all the herbs, the hot peppers (if using) and the apple cider vinegar in a pint-size (473-ml) jar. Cover the jar with a lid and put it in a cool, dark place to infuse for 4 to 6 weeks. Strain out the herbs when ready to use and stir in the honey (if using).

Take 1 tablespoon (15 ml) whenever you feel a sickness coming on, up to 3 times daily. It can also be taken once or twice daily throughout cold and flu season as a preventative measure and to help boost your overall immunity. It can be taken straight or stirred into water.

This vinegar infusion, with the hot peppers omitted, is safe for children ages 2 and older. Please follow the dosage guidelines on page 23 and use diluted in water.

Tip: Other possible additions include sliced fresh horseradish, a sprig of fresh rosemary, fresh sage leaves or dried astragalus root.

OREGANO-INFUSED OIL WITH LEMON

When the threat of winter sickness is around, oregano-infused oil can be immensely helpful. Fresh oregano is full of antioxidants and is antibacterial, making it one of the most healthful herbs in your garden. It also has powerful antimicrobial actions, making it usable as a natural topical sanitizer. This is the only infused oil in this book that I call for using fresh herbal material, as normally dried herbs are used to help keep the oil from becoming rancid. The addition of lemon juice will help it keep longer, and will also increase the acidity enough to make an unfavorable environment for botulism.

Yield: about ¾ cup (180 ml)

Ingredients
1 cup (11 g) loosely packed fresh oregano sprigs

¾ cup (180 ml) extra-virgin olive oil

2 tbsp (30 ml) lemon juice

Instructions
Combine the oregano, olive oil and lemon juice in a half-pint (236-ml) jar. Because this oil infusion uses fresh herbs, it's important to make sure that the oil completely covers the oregano. Cover the jar with a lid and shake to combine. Put in a cool, dark place to infuse for 4 to 6 weeks. Strain out the oregano with a fine-mesh sieve when ready to use, and be sure to use up the oil within a month.

One tablespoon (15 ml) can be taken daily as a preventative measure and immune system booster, or twice per day at the first sign of illness to help speed recovery. It can also be used topically as an antimicrobial agent and natural sanitizer. Rub a thin layer on the hands to help disinfect and sanitize.

This oil infusion is safe for children ages 2 and older. Please follow the dosage guidelines on page 23.

Tip: This oregano-infused oil also has wonderful culinary uses! Serve it alongside some crusty bread for dipping, or brush it on grilled veggies or meat.

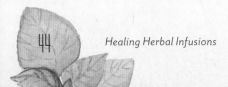

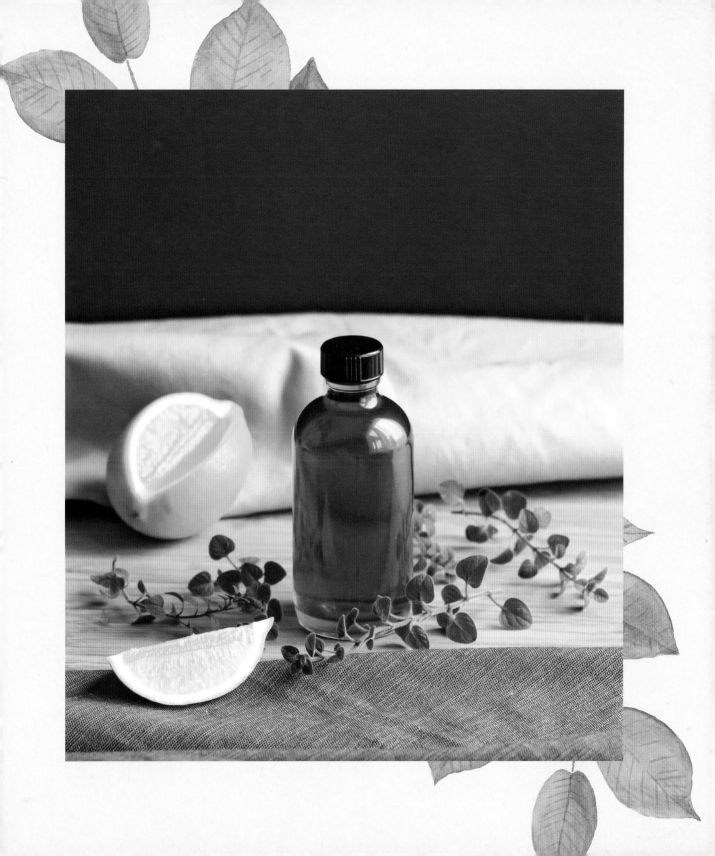

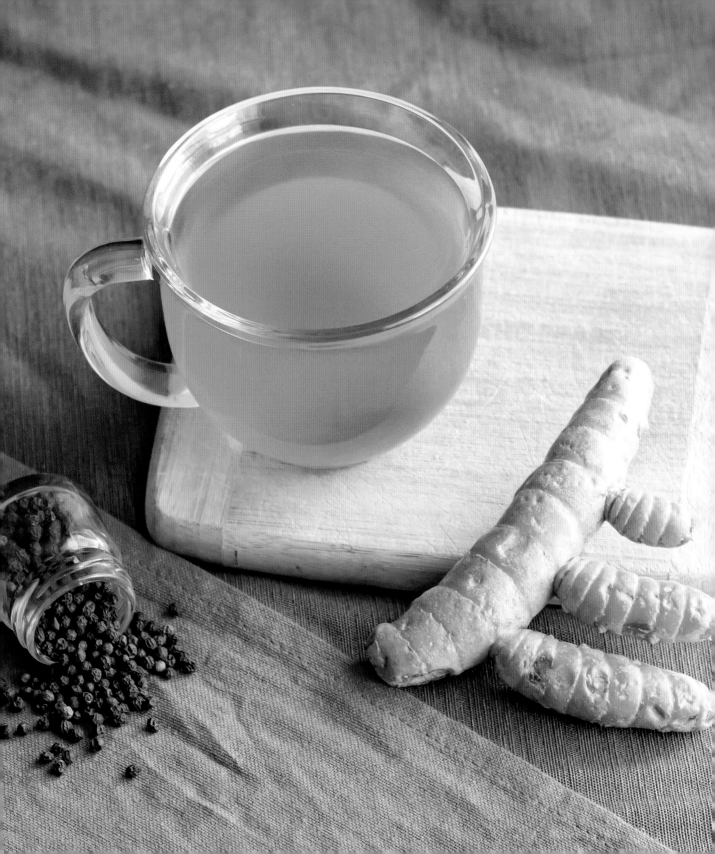

INFUSIONS TO SOOTHE YOUR ACHES & PAINS

Herbs are there for us when we need them, and many have wonderful healing abilities for our everyday aches and pains. Arnica helps sore muscles and bruising. Lavender and peppermint are calming and good for aching muscles. And calendula, plantain and yarrow are superstars at healing minor cuts, burns, bug bites and wounds. Infusing these herbs into oils is a great way to use their benefits; either use the oils as is or turn them into balms and salves.

Powerful pain-relieving and inflammation-reducing herbs, such as white willow, birch bark, basil, thyme and turmeric, are also great to have around for making teas that ease troublesome aches and stiffness. Cannabis is making itself well known in recent years as an herbal ally for chronic pain. With these herbs and remedies by your side, you will be feeling pain-free in no time.

47

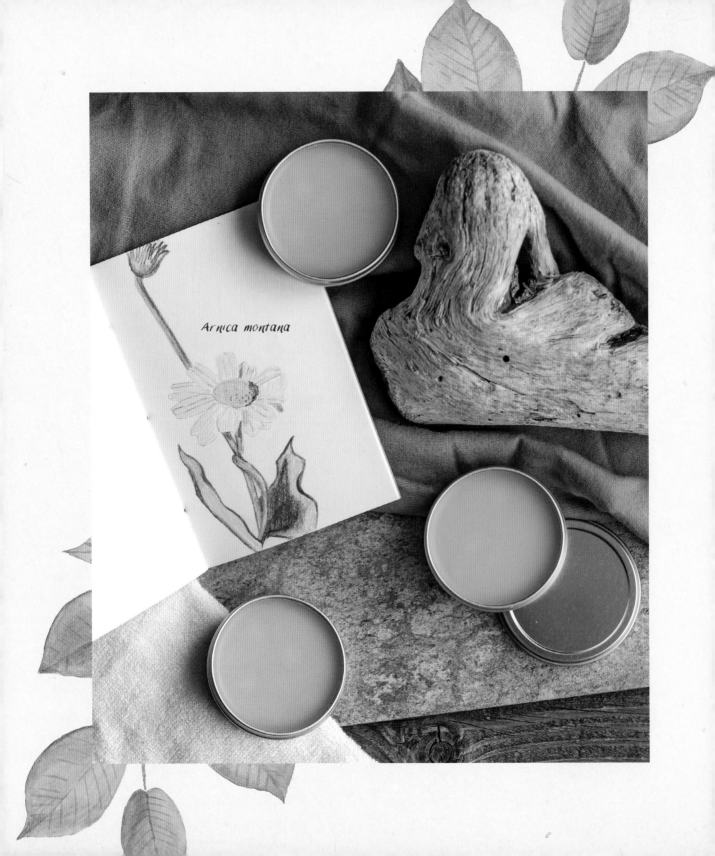

Arnica montana

ARNICA SALVE FOR SPRAINS & BRUISES

Arnica montana is a yellow mountain flower that is particularly good at relieving the pain associated with sore muscles, sprains, strains and bruises. It has powerful anti-inflammatory properties that rival over-the-counter painkillers, all wrapped up in one pretty flower. This salve is a great way to easily apply arnica, and as an added benefit, it is also wonderful for your skin. A word of caution: Arnica is toxic when taken internally, so it should only be used topically and on unbroken skin, and it should never be ingested. Because of this, it should be stored well out of reach of children and pets.

Yield: about 5 ounces (150 ml) of salve

Ingredients

For the Infused Oil
½ cup (5 g) loosely packed dried arnica flowers
¼ cup (60 ml) coconut oil, melted
¼ cup (60 ml) olive oil
¼ cup (60 ml) sweet almond oil

For the Salve
½ cup (120 ml) arnica-infused oil
½ oz (14 g) beeswax
½ oz (14 g) shea butter

Instructions

Combine the arnica flowers with the coconut, olive and sweet almond oils in a half-pint (236-ml) jar. Cover the jar with a lid and shake to mix well. Put the jar in a cool, dark place to infuse for 4 to 6 weeks.

When you are ready to make the salve, strain the flowers from the oil using a fine-mesh sieve. If the coconut oil has solidified in the oil infusion, gently heat it by setting the jar in a pan of warm water to melt the oil before straining. Measure out ½ cup (120 ml) of the infused oil. Put the oil into a double boiler on medium heat (see tips for making your own double boiler on page 20). Add the beeswax to the oil and continue to heat until it has completely melted. Next, add the shea butter, and when it has melted, remove the mixture from the heat. Carefully pour the mixture into jars or tins. Let the salve cool and set up for 3 to 4 hours before use.

Apply the salve on sore muscles, sprains, strains and bruises as often as needed for several days, or until the pain has subsided.

This arnica salve is safe to use on children ages 8 and older following a patch test (see page 23). For those under the age of 8, I recommend using Boo-Boo Balm (page 182) instead.

Tip: Other pain-relieving herbs you can use are Saint John's wort, cayenne and peppermint.

CANNABIS-INFUSED COCONUT OIL FOR BODY ACHES

With the laws in the United States starting to relax a bit on medical cannabis, it's becoming a popular choice for relieving all types of aches and pains, from a pulled muscle to chronic pain and everything in between. There are two main compounds in cannabis that provide medicinal benefit: THC, which is the same compound that has mind-altering effects when inhaled or ingested, and CBD, which is particularly good for pain control. I use the stovetop method for heating this infused oil; it facilitates a process called "decarboxylation" that makes the medicinal compounds in cannabis more bioavailable. When using medical cannabis topically, it makes sense to find a variety that is high in CBD, then it's up to you whether you want a lower or higher THC level. Some good CBD varieties are Charlotte's Web, Harlequin and ACDC. Contact your local cannabis pharmacy for more information on which strain is best for your needs. Please check all of your local laws before using cannabis as medicine to be sure that it is legal in your area.

Yield: about 1 cup (240 ml)

Ingredients
¼–½ cup (5–10 g) dried cannabis buds or trimmings

1 cup (240 ml) coconut oil

Instructions
Place the cannabis and coconut oil in a small saucepan and heat on low for 4 to 8 hours. The longer you heat it, the stronger the final oil will be. Be careful that the oil doesn't become too hot to avoid burning the cannabis, aiming to keep the temperature less than 150°F (65°C). Strain out the plant material through a fine-mesh sieve and store the oil in a jar. It will solidify at room temperature (below 76°F [24°C]), but will melt on contact with the skin.

Rub on sore muscles, joints or other painful areas as often as needed for relief.

I do not recommend using this cannabis infusion on children under the age of 18.

Tip: This cannabis oil can also be made into a salve by melting 1 ounce (28 g) of beeswax into 1 cup (240 ml) of the strained infused oil over a double boiler, and then pouring into tins or jars.

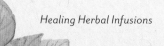

Healing Herbal Infusions

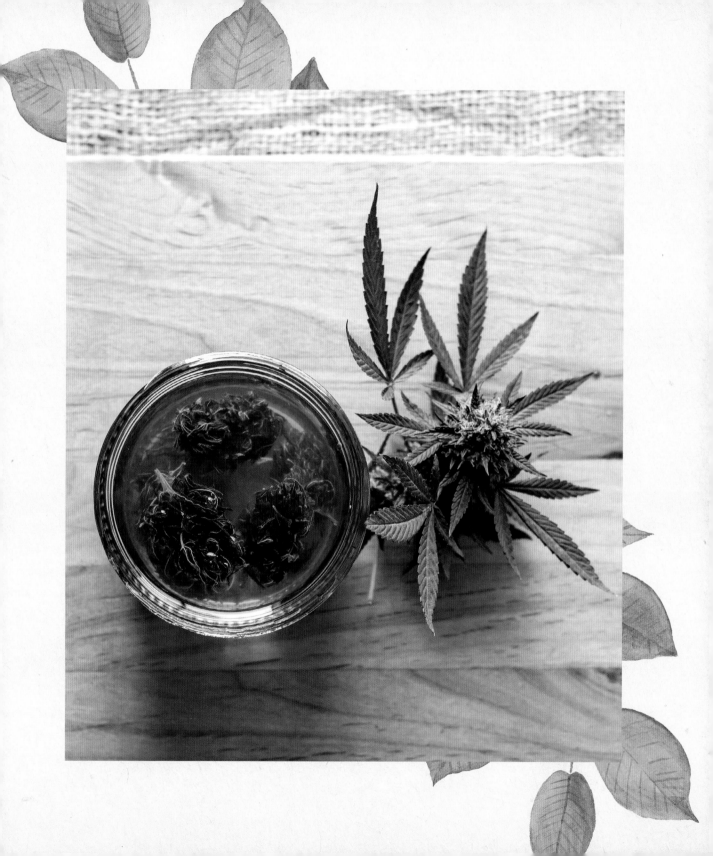

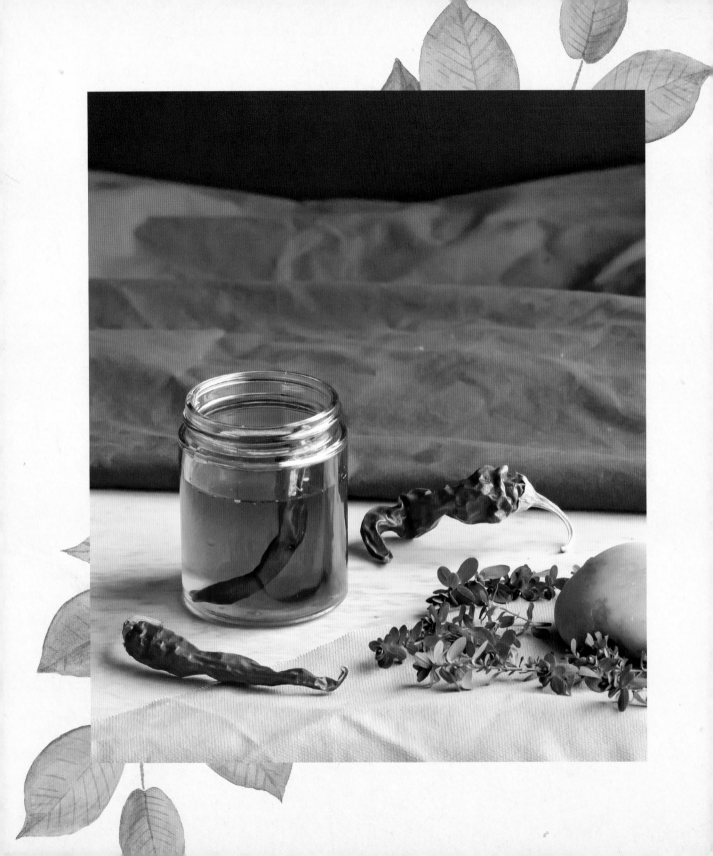

SAINT JOHN'S WORT & CAYENNE WARMING OIL

Saint John's wort has become a popular home remedy for mood and depression (see page 131 for a mood-elevating Saint John's wort tincture recipe). It is less known for its ability to soothe sore muscles and painful joints. When you add the warming effects of cayenne, this infused oil becomes a highly effective topical and highly localized pain reliever. If you have sensitive skin, do a patch test first to make sure that you won't have a reaction to the spicy pepper. Feel free to leave out the cayenne if you'd like—Saint John's wort has immense healing benefits on its own.

Yield: about ¾ cup (180 ml)

Ingredients
⅓ cup (20 g) dried or ⅔ cup (40 g) fresh Saint John's wort flowers and leaves
1 small dried cayenne pepper
½ cup (120 ml) olive oil
¼ cup (60 ml) coconut oil, melted

Instructions
If you are using dried Saint John's wort flowers, combine them and the cayenne pepper with the olive and coconut oils in a half-pint (236-ml) jar. Cover the jar with a lid and shake to mix well. Put the jar in a cool, dark place to infuse for 4 to 6 weeks. Strain out the plant material and cayenne pepper with a fine-mesh sieve before using. If the coconut oil has solidified in the oil infusion, gently heat it by setting the jar in a pan of warm water to melt the oil before straining.

If you choose to use fresh Saint John's wort flowers, please follow the instructions for the heat method of infusing oils on page 17, and be sure to use up the oil within a month.

Rub the oil on sore muscles and joints as needed for pain relief.

This oil infusion, with the cayenne omitted, is safe to use on children ages 2 and older following a patch test (see page 23).

Tip: This warming oil can also be made into a salve if you prefer. Simply melt ½ ounce (14 g) of beeswax into ½ cup (120 ml) of the strained infused oil in a double boiler, and then pour into tins or jars.

LAVENDER & PEPPERMINT SORE MUSCLE OIL

We all get a little bit of soreness and stiffness from time to time, whether it's from going on a long and strenuous hike or working all day out in the garden. Luckily, you have pain-relieving lavender and peppermint on your side! This is the oil to turn to for sore muscles due to overexertion. After soaking your tired muscles in a hot bath, rub this infused oil on them to help relieve the soreness. As an added benefit, you will also smell amazing!

Yield: about ¾ cup (180 ml)

Ingredients
¼ cup (8 g) dried lavender flowers
¼ cup (8 g) dried peppermint
½ cup (120 ml) coconut oil, melted
¼ cup (60 ml) sweet almond oil
5–10 drops lavender essential oil (optional, see note)
5–10 drops peppermint essential oil (optional, see note)

Instructions
Combine the lavender and peppermint with the coconut and sweet almond oils in a half-pint (236-ml) jar. Cover the jar with a lid and shake to mix well. Put the jar in a cool, dark place to infuse for 4 to 6 weeks. Strain out the plant material with a fine-mesh sieve. If the coconut oil has solidified in the oil infusion, gently heat it by setting the jar in a pan of warm water to melt the oil before straining. Add in the essential oils (if using) and stir well.

Rub the oil on sore muscles and joints as needed for pain relief.

This oil infusion is safe to use on children ages 2 and older following a patch test (see page 23).

Note: Omit the essential oils for those under age 13.

Tip: Lavender and peppermint are also both effective for easing headache pain. Try rubbing a bit of this infused oil on your temples or behind your ears for some relief.

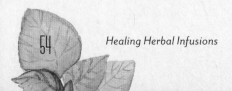

Healing Herbal Infusions

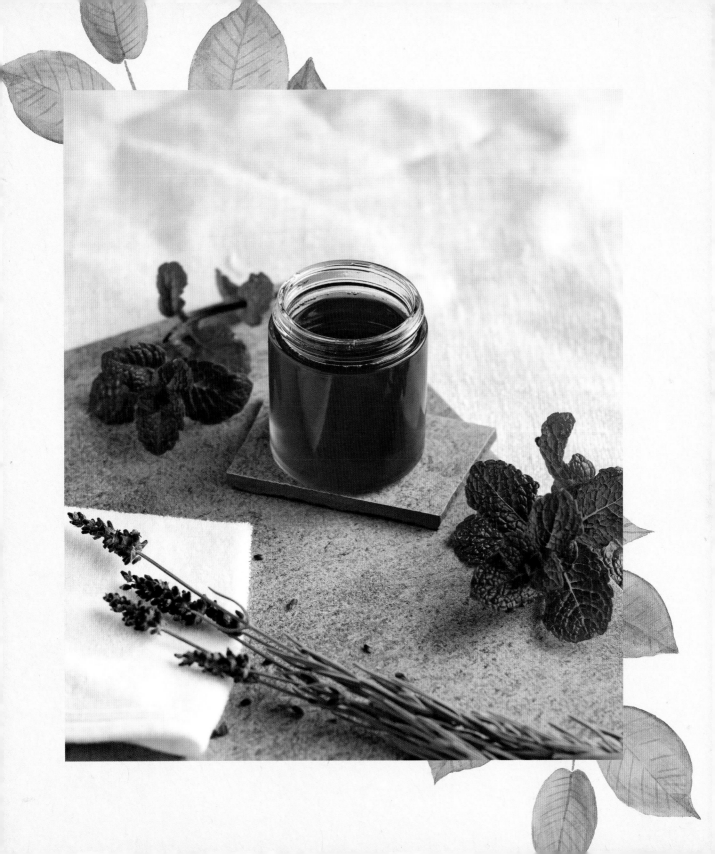

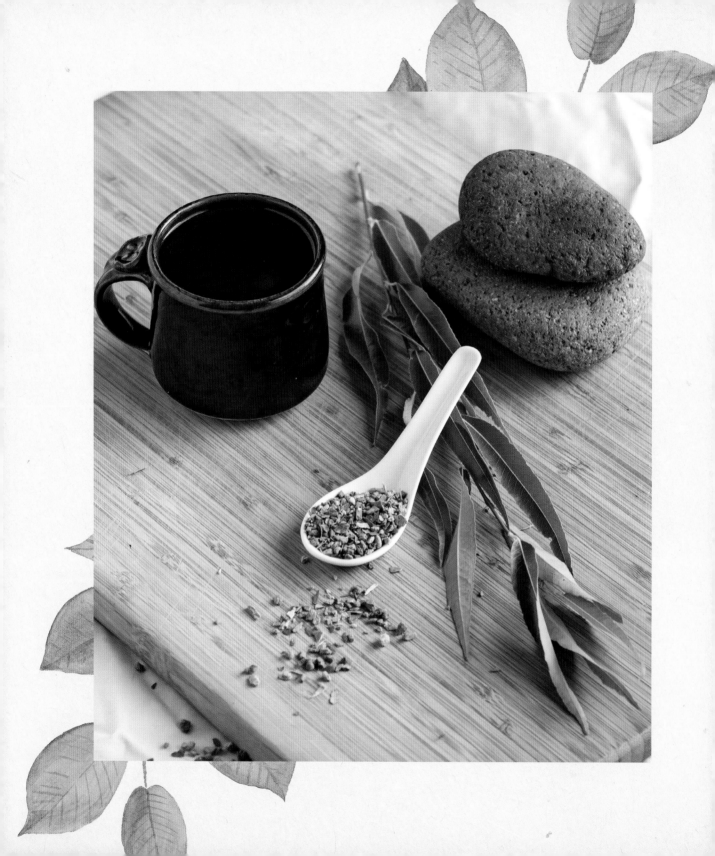

WHITE WILLOW & BIRCH BARK TEA FOR PAIN RELIEF

Many over-the-counter and prescription medications have their roots in plant medicine. White willow bark is one of those, as one of its main components—salicylic acid—is where aspirin was originally derived. Birch bark also contains some salicylic acid, and it has a nice, aromatic, wintergreen-like flavor that makes this tea pleasant to drink. Using the whole herb rather than just a single component gives you more benefits from flavonoids and other natural compounds, and it also eliminates the harshness on the stomach that aspirin can have. Be aware that this tea will have a mild blood-thinning effect, just like regular aspirin, so avoid drinking it if that is a concern. It should also be avoided by pregnant and nursing women, and children under the age of 18.

Yield: 2 cups (480 ml)

Ingredients
2 cups (480 ml) water
2 tbsp (8 g) white willow bark or twigs, broken into small pieces
1 tbsp (6 g) birch bark or twigs, broken into small pieces

Instructions
Bring the water to a boil and pour over the white willow and birch bark. Let the infusion steep for 10 to 15 minutes, then strain out the bark before drinking. For a stronger tea, follow the directions on page 15 for a long or overnight infusion or decoction.

Drink 1 to 2 cups (240 to 480 ml) throughout the day to help relieve acute pain and inflammation. Do not take for more than 1 to 2 weeks at a time.

I do not recommend children under the age of 18, or pregnant or nursing women, take this tea.

Tip: Both white willow and birch trees are relatively easy to forage for, so grab your guidebook and be on the lookout for nature's aspirin! White willow grows in abundance almost everywhere, and shavings of the bark or small twigs can be taken safely without any concern of hurting the plant. Birch bark and small twigs should only be taken from dead and dying trees so as not to hurt or inhibit the growth of healthy trees. Trim off the outer bark, as the inner bark has the most benefits.

BASIL, THYME & OREGANO TEA FOR CHRONIC PAIN

Having an herb garden in your backyard, or even in a sunny windowsill inside, has more benefits than just for use in cooking. Most of your regular garden herbs are also highly medicinal, so it makes sense to have them close at hand! Basil, thyme and oregano all have pain- and inflammation-reducing properties, and they make a wonderful and highly drinkable tea. I recommend using fresh herbs in this mix, organic if possible. Even if you don't grow them, they should be easy enough to find at your local market. Pregnant women should avoid using large amounts of basil.

Yield: 2 cups (480 ml)

Ingredients
2 cups (480 ml) water
½ cup (8 g) loosely packed mix of roughly chopped fresh basil, thyme and oregano

---

Instructions
Bring the water to a boil and pour over the fresh herbs in a pint-size (473-ml) mason jar. Let the infusion steep for 10 to 15 minutes, then strain out the herbs before drinking. For a stronger tea, follow the directions on page 15 for a long or overnight infusion.

Drink daily, as often as needed, to help relieve chronic pain and inflammation. It may take several weeks of daily use for the pain to subside.

This tea is safe for children ages 2 and older. Please follow the dosage guidelines on page 23.

Tip: All three of these herbs are also great for the immune system, so drink this tea when you feel a sickness coming on to help you get better quickly!

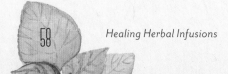

Healing Herbal Infusions

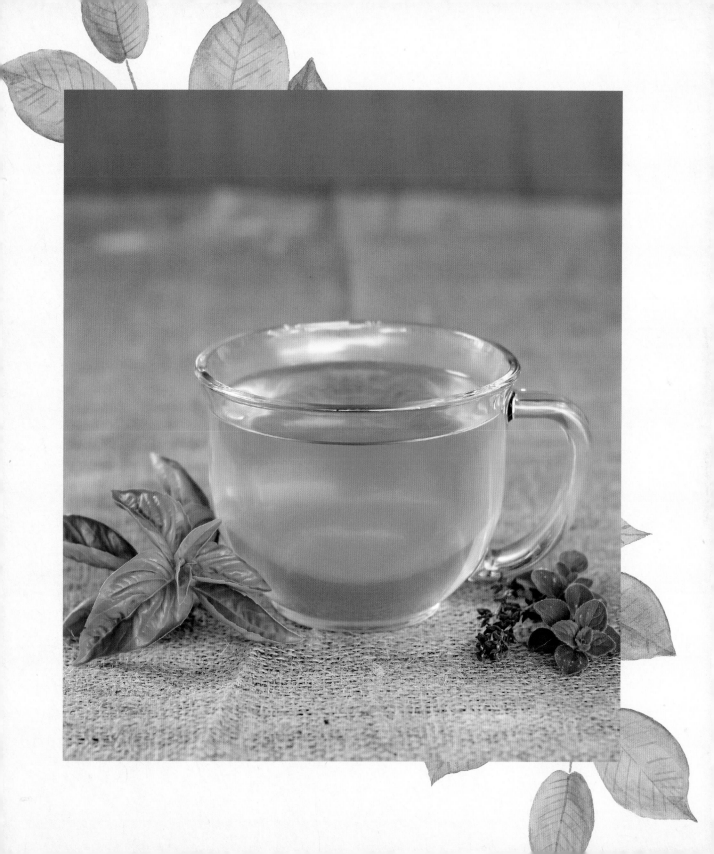

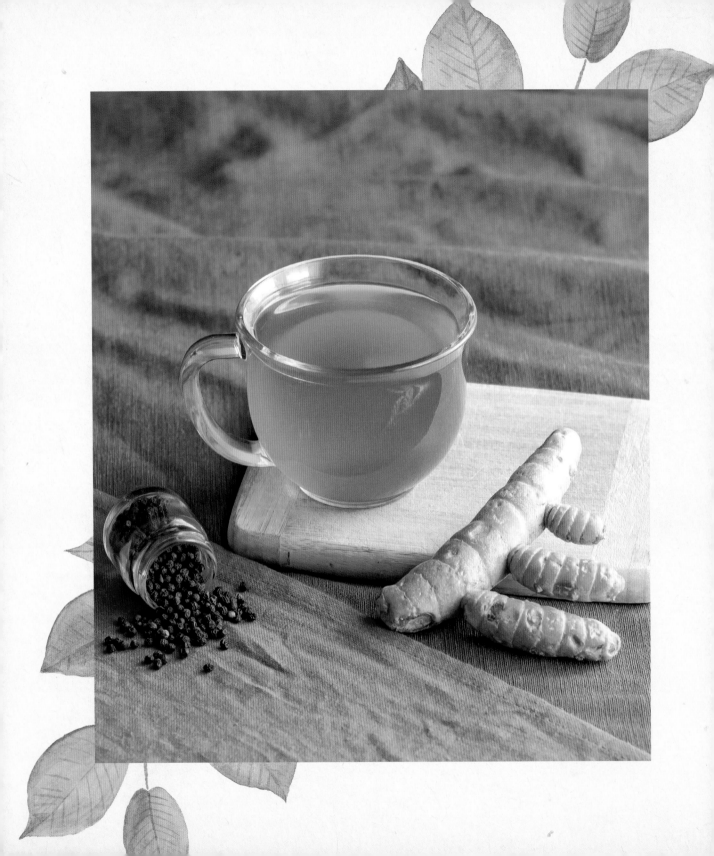

TURMERIC & BLACK PEPPER TEA FOR CHRONIC INFLAMMATION

Turmeric has become an important herbal ally in recent years, especially for those who have excess inflammation, such as arthritis, irritable bowel syndrome or old sports injuries. Turmeric root is in the same family as the more commonly found ginger and is a powerful natural anti-inflammatory. One problem is that curcumin, the main compound in turmeric that gives it these benefits, isn't easily absorbed by the body. Luckily, that is an easy fix, as the piperine in black pepper makes it more bioavailable. I have fond memories of drinking turmeric tea in Costa Rica on my honeymoon, and whenever I see fresh turmeric in the grocery store, I pick some up to make a cup of this warming tea!

Yield: 2 cups (480 ml)

Ingredients
¾ cup (75 g) sliced fresh turmeric
2 tsp (6 g) whole black peppercorns
2½ cups (600 ml) water

Instructions
Combine the turmeric, peppercorns and water in a small saucepan. Bring to a boil. Boil for 10 to 15 minutes, then remove the pan from the heat and let sit to slightly cool for several minutes. Strain out the turmeric and peppercorns when ready to use. Be forewarned that fresh turmeric can stain your cooking utensils, hands and clothing a bright orange color that can be hard to remove.

Drink 1 to 2 cups (240 to 480 ml) per day to help reduce chronic inflammation.

This tea is safe for children ages 2 and older. Please follow the dosage guidelines on page 23.

Tip: Turmeric milk (also called golden milk) is a staple of Ayurvedic medicine and is a great way to get a dose of turmeric. Replace the water with milk (nondairy milk also works), add the turmeric and black peppercorns and warm on low in a saucepan for 10 to 15 minutes. Stir in a spoonful or two of raw honey, if desired, for a yummy medicinal drink!

FOUR-HERB WOUND SALVE

This is a recipe that I formulated many years ago, and it is one that I use time and time again. These four herbs each have unique benefits for minor cuts and scrapes on their own, and when combined, they make for a potent wound healer. Yarrow stops the bleeding; plantain is soothing and prevents infections; comfrey helps new skin cells grow; and calendula speeds healing and reduces scarring. One thing to note is that this salve should only be used on minor wounds. Anything deep or potentially requiring stitches should be seen by a doctor.

Yield: about 5 ounces (150 ml) of salve

Ingredients

For the Infused Oil
2 tbsp (3 g) dried calendula flowers
2 tbsp (5 g) dried yarrow flowers
2 tbsp (5 g) dried plantain leaf
2 tbsp (5 g) dried comfrey leaf
¼ cup (60 ml) coconut oil, melted

¼ cup (60 ml) olive oil
¼ cup (60 ml) sweet almond oil

For the Salve
½ cup (120 ml) four-herb-infused oil
½ oz (14 g) beeswax

Instructions

Combine the calendula, yarrow, plantain and comfrey with the coconut, olive and sweet almond oils in a half-pint (236-ml) jar. Cover the jar with a lid and shake to mix well. Put the jar in a cool, dark place to infuse for 4 to 6 weeks.

When you are ready to make the salve, strain the herbs from the oil using a fine-mesh sieve. If the coconut oil has solidified in the oil infusion, gently heat it by setting the jar in a pan of warm water to melt the oil before straining. Measure out ½ cup (120 ml) of the infused oil, saving any excess oil for later use if you wish. Put the oil into a double boiler on medium heat (see tips for making your own double boiler on page 20). Add the beeswax to the oil and continue to heat until all of the beeswax has completely melted. Carefully pour the mixture into jars or tins. Let the salve cool and set up for 3 to 4 hours before use.

Apply it on minor cuts, scrapes and wounds as needed to help speed healing.

This wound salve is safe to use on children ages 13 and older following a patch test (see page 23). For those under the age of 13, I recommend using Boo-Boo Balm (page 182) instead.

Tip: You can also use this salve on rashes, bug bites, bruises, minor burns, blemishes and scars.

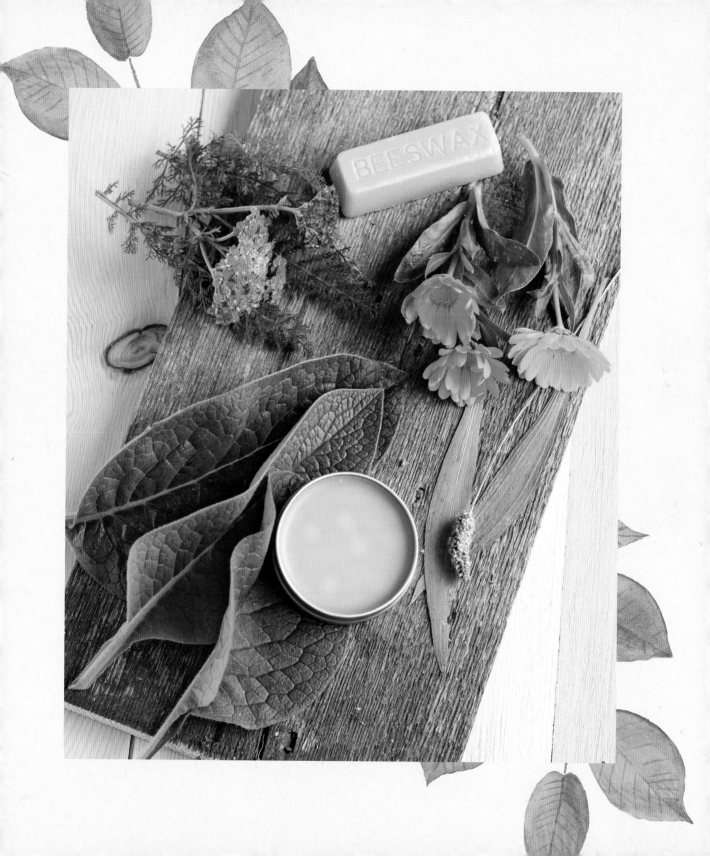

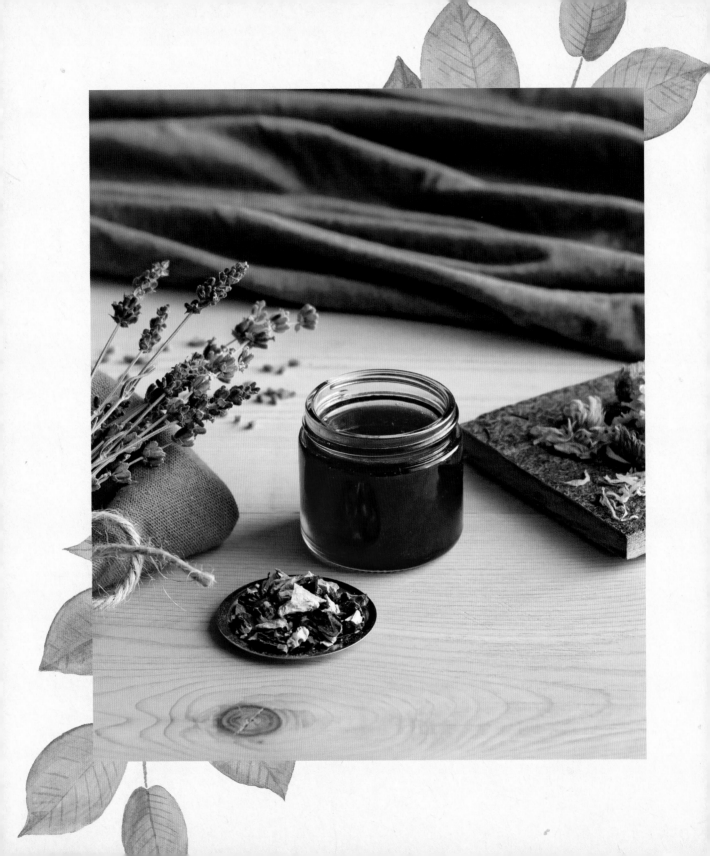

HERBAL HONEY BURN OINTMENT

Burns can be tricky to treat, and one thing to keep in mind is that you don't want to use anything oil based, as it can seal in the heat. That means that traditional infused oils and salves aren't ideal, although they can be helpful once the healing process is underway. Honey is soothing for burns, as well as being antibacterial. It makes for a wonderful natural burn ointment when combined with healing herbs and a small amount of coconut oil and apple cider vinegar. Lavender is especially amazing for treating burns! For second- or third-degree burns, please consult your doctor before using this remedy.

Yield: about ¾ cup (180 ml)

Ingredients
¼ cup (5 g) dried calendula flowers

2 tbsp (5 g) dried lavender flowers

1 tbsp (7 g) dried comfrey root

½ cup (120 ml) raw honey

2 tbsp (30 ml) coconut oil, melted

2 tbsp (30 ml) raw apple cider vinegar

Instructions
Combine the calendula, lavender and comfrey root in a half-pint (236-ml) jar, then add the honey, coconut oil and apple cider vinegar. Stir well to combine, then cover the jar and place it in a cool, dark place to infuse for 4 to 6 weeks, stirring every so often. Strain out the herbs with a fine-mesh sieve before using.

Apply a small amount to a minor burn several times daily for relief and to speed healing.

This burn ointment is safe to use on children ages 13 and older following a patch test (see page 23). For use on children under the age of 13, omit the comfrey root and then it is safe to use for ages 1 and older.

Tip: This burn ointment also works very well on minor cuts, scrapes, bug bites and rashes.

ITCHY BITE & STING BALM

When the inevitable bites and stings of summertime happen, plantain is your herbal friend! It is soothing and will stop the itch almost immediately. In fact, if you do happen to get bit or stung, look around for a plantain leaf—they are easy to identify and grow almost everywhere. Chew it up and apply directly to the affected area. It will ease the pain on contact and the healing process will begin. It's handy to make this balm in tubes so that you can easily stash them in your daypack, first aid kit or with your camping gear. Start the infused oil for this balm in the springtime so that you're prepared for summertime bug bites!

Yield: about 5 ounces (150 ml) of balm

Ingredients

For the Infused Oil
¼ cup (10 g) dried plantain leaf
2 tbsp (4 g) dried chickweed
2 tbsp (5 g) dried lavender flowers
¼ cup (60 ml) coconut oil, melted
¼ cup (60 ml) olive oil
¼ cup (60 ml) sweet almond oil

For the Balm
½ cup (120 ml) herb-infused oil
½ oz (14 g) beeswax (double the amount if using tubes)
½ oz (14 g) shea butter

Instructions

Combine the plantain, chickweed and lavender with the coconut, olive and sweet almond oils in a half-pint (236-ml) jar. Cover the jar with a lid and shake to mix well. Put the jar in a cool, dark place to infuse for 4 to 6 weeks.

When you are ready to make the balm, strain the herbs from the oil using a fine-mesh sieve. If the coconut oil has solidified in the oil infusion, gently heat it by setting the jar in a pan of warm water to melt the oil before straining. Measure out ½ cup (120 ml) of the infused oil, saving any excess oil for later use if you wish. Put the oil into a double boiler on medium heat (see tips for making your own double boiler on page 20). Add the beeswax to the oil and continue to heat until all of the beeswax has completely melted. Next, add the shea butter, and when it has melted, remove the mixture from the heat. Carefully pour the mixture into jars, tins or tubes. Let the balm cool and set up for 3 to 4 hours before use.

Apply as often as needed to relieve the itch and discomfort from bug bites and stings.

This bite and sting balm is safe to use on children ages 6 months and older following a patch test (see page 23).

Healing Herbal Infusions

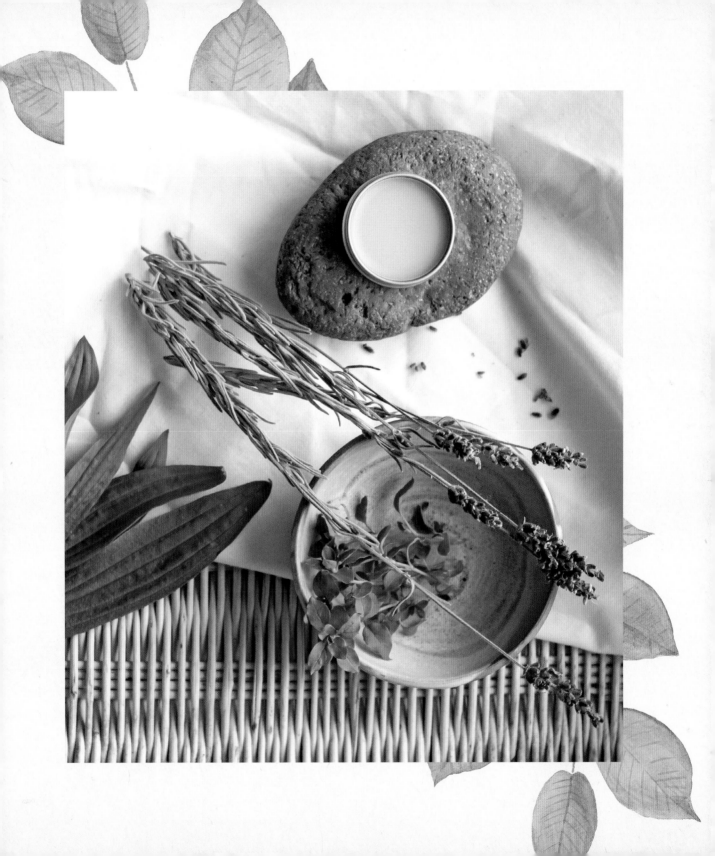

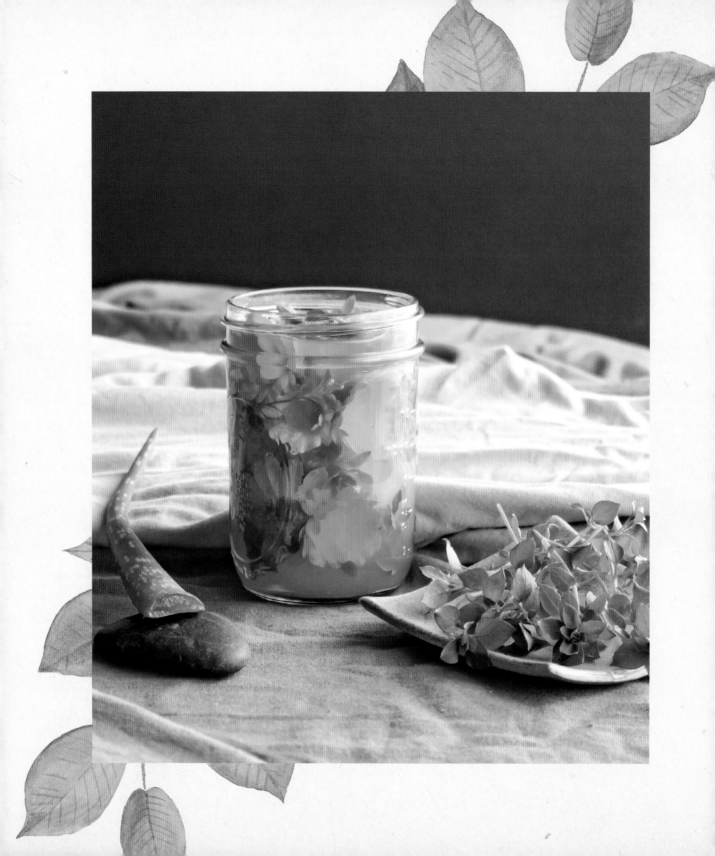

... soothing and cooling down sunburns. The pure gel ...ouple of fresh herbs makes it even more beneficial. ... chickweed is mucilaginous, which means it provides ...o use fresh calendula and chickweed in this infusion, ... If you have access to large amounts of fresh aloe ...d scrape out the gel, then process in a blender for a ...ing a minimally processed prepared aloe vera gel for ...that you're prepared for summer sunburns!

rs

...ra gel in a pint-size (473-ml) jar. Cover the jar with a lid ...l, dark place to infuse for 3 to 4 weeks. Strain out the ... infusion is best stored in the refrigerator to extend its ...t when applied to sunburned skin. It will last for about

...eal sunburns.

...6 months and older following a patch test (see page 23).

...nedicinal houseplant to have around. If you don't have ...break off a leaf and rub the cut side on a sunburn for

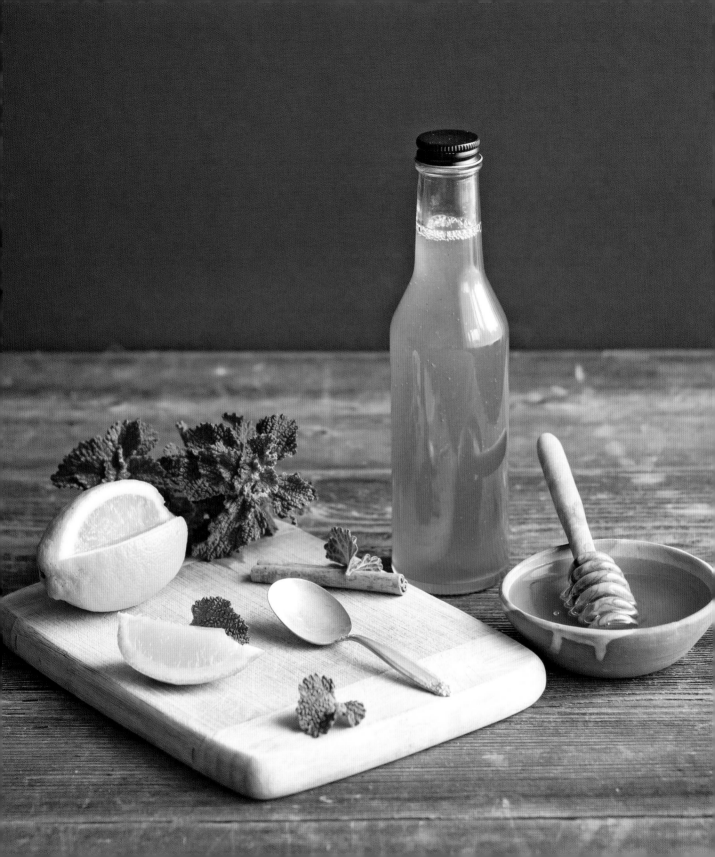

INFUSIONS TO RELIEVE WHAT AILS YOU

We all have ailments that rear their head from time to time, some more serious than others. When there is an issue that flares up, many times turning to herbs is a good solution. Headaches, toothaches, earaches, sore throats, urinary tract infections and eczema are all common problems that can benefit from herbal medicine. Thankfully, there are some amazing health-promoting herbs that can help us with these discomforts in a safe way, often without having to resort to taking prescription medication. Lemon balm, a plant that grows nearly everywhere and in abundance, can reduce headaches and heal cold sores. Yarrow is a highly effective fever reducer, whether used internally or externally. Common sage and horehound can soothe a sore throat fast. Uva ursi, also known as kinnikinnick or bearberry, not only relieves and heals a urinary tract infection but can prevent it from reoccurring. For every ailment, there is an herb that can help!

71

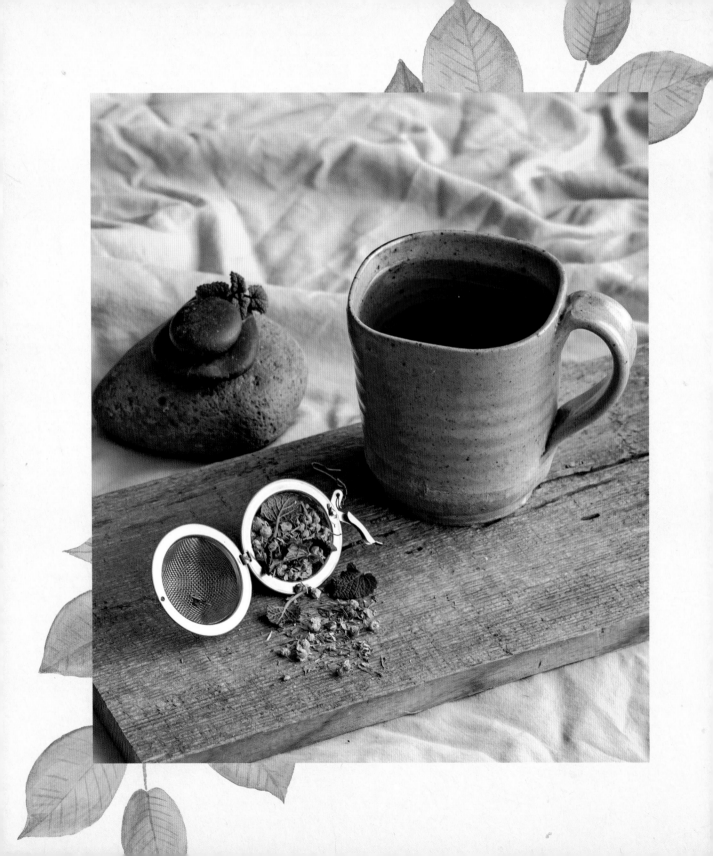

HEADACHE RELIEF TEA

Everyone gets a headache from time to time, and they are no fun. Luckily, there are herbs that are quite effective in helping to relieve the pain from headaches. Skullcap is particularly good at this. It also calms the nerves that could be the cause of the headache to begin with. Lemon balm and chamomile are relaxing and can help to take the pressure off. Brew up a hot mug of this tea, get cozy and sip your headache away!

Yield: 2 cups (480 ml)

Ingredients
2 cups (480 ml) water
2 tbsp (3 g) dried skullcap
1 tbsp (1 g) dried lemon balm
1 tbsp (1 g) dried chamomile flowers

Instructions
Bring the water to a boil and pour over the dried herbs. Let the infusion steep for 10 to 15 minutes, then strain out the herbs before drinking.

Drink 1 to 2 cups (240 to 480 ml), sipping throughout the duration of a headache to help ease the pain.

This tea is safe for children ages 2 and older. Please follow the dosage guidelines on page 23.

Tip: Skullcap is a plant in the mint family that can be wildcrafted in certain areas. Besides easing headache pain, it is also often used to relieve stress, anxiety and muscle tension.

FEVERFEW MIGRAINE PREVENTATIVE TINCTURE

If you are someone who suffers from migraines, you've probably tried everything to alleviate that horrible pain and pressure when you feel one coming on. While this feverfew tincture may not be able to get rid of that pain once it's already settled in, what it can do is help to prevent more migraines from coming on. It needs to be taken regularly for 2 to 3 months before these effects can be noticed. Feverfew is very easy to grow and has pretty little daisy-like flowers, which makes it a nice addition to any medicinal herb garden. Pregnant women should avoid using feverfew.

Yield: about ¾ cup (180 ml)

Ingredients
1 cup (21 g) loosely packed whole, fresh feverfew flowers and leaves
¾ cup (180 ml) vodka or other neutral spirits

Instructions
Combine the feverfew and spirits in a half-pint (236-ml) jar, then cover with a lid. Put the jar in a cool, dark place to infuse for 4 to 6 weeks. When ready to use, strain out the herbs with a fine-mesh sieve. Store the tincture in small bottles with droppers for easy use.

Take 1 teaspoon (5 ml) daily as a migraine preventative.

For children and those wishing to avoid alcohol, this tincture can be made with vegetable glycerine instead of the neutral spirits. If made in this manner, it is safe for children ages 2 and older. Please follow the dosage guidelines on page 23.

Tip: Beyond migraines, feverfew is also great for regular headaches. Combine it in a tea with lemon balm and lavender to help relieve the pain.

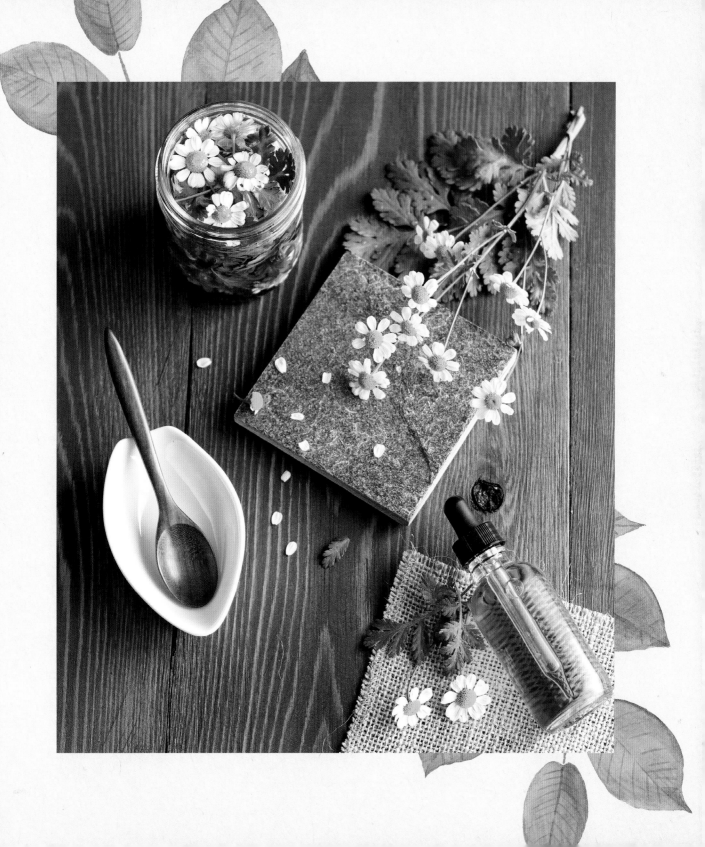

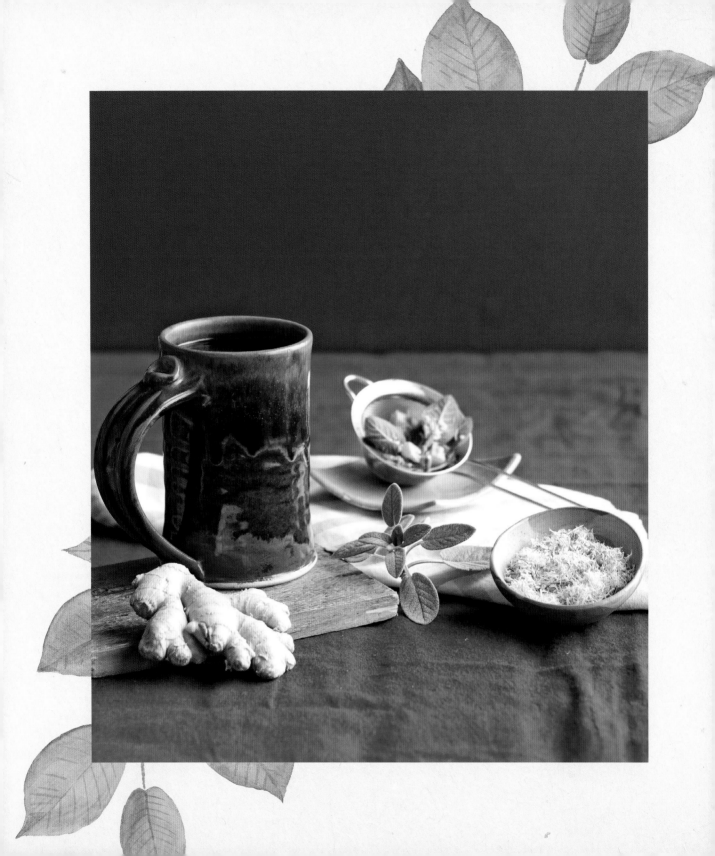

SAGE, MARSHMALLOW & GINGER SORE THROAT TEA

A sore throat can be really uncomfortable, and sometimes a cup of hot tea is the only thing that sounds tolerable. Sage is particularly alleviating for sore throats, with antibacterial and anti-inflammatory properties. Marshmallow root adds a soothing mucilaginous quality that helps to mitigate the pain, and ginger is a tried-and-true remedy for preventing and relieving many cold and flu symptoms. A little bit of honey and lemon, if you so desire, will make this a potent and delicious-tasting tea that will help your throat feel better in no time. Sage should be avoided by nursing women as it can reduce your supply. Thyme or oregano are both good alternatives with similar benefits.

Yield: 2 cups (480 ml)

Ingredients
2½ cups (600 ml) water
½ cup (8 g) loosely packed, roughly chopped, fresh sage leaves
1 tbsp (2 g) dried marshmallow root
1-inch (2.5-cm) piece fresh ginger, sliced
Honey and/or lemon, to taste (optional)

Instructions
Bring the water to a boil and pour it over the herbs. Let the infusion steep for 10 to 15 minutes, then strain out the herbs before drinking. Add a spoonful or two of honey and a squeeze of lemon, if desired.

Drink 1 to 2 cups (240 to 480 ml) as often as needed to help ease the pain from a dry, sore or scratchy throat.

This tea is safe for children ages 2 and older. Please follow the dosage guidelines on page 23.

Tip: Sage is a perennial herb that is easy to grow and stays hardy and evergreen to well-below-freezing temperatures. I always make sure to have at least one sage plant growing in my garden so that I have access to its medicinal and culinary benefits year-round.

HOREHOUND SORE THROAT SYRUP

A dry, scratchy sore throat is often the first sign of a cold coming on, and sometimes it will persist for days. Instead of taking sugary over-the-counter sore throat syrups, make this one at home using horehound instead. Horehound is a bitter herb that has been used for ages for treating sore throats and coughs, often in the form of "horehound candy." Slippery elm is mucilaginous and very soothing on an inflamed and sore throat. Honey tames horehound's bitterness and helps to coat the throat and ease the pain. Orange peel and cinnamon improve the flavor to make it a bit more palatable.

Yield: about 2 cups (480 ml)

Ingredients
1 cup (18 g) loosely packed fresh horehound cuttings

¼ cup (10 g) dried slippery elm

1 tbsp (8 g) dried orange peel

1 cinnamon stick

2 cups (480 ml) water

1 cup (240 ml) raw honey

Instructions
Combine the horehound, slippery elm, orange peel, cinnamon stick and water in a small saucepan. Bring to a boil, then reduce the heat and simmer for about 20 minutes, or until the liquid has reduced by half. Remove the pan from the heat and let cool to room temperature. Strain out the herbs with a fine-mesh sieve, then stir in the honey. Store the syrup in a covered jar in the refrigerator and it will keep for 2 to 4 weeks. If you'd like to increase the shelf life of this syrup, freeze it in baggies or ice cube trays and then thaw as needed before use.

Take 1 tablespoon (15 ml) every 2 hours as needed to help ease a sore throat.

This syrup is safe for children ages 2 and older. Please follow the dosage guidelines on page 23.

Tip: Slippery elm is considered an at-risk herb due to unethical overharvesting, so I try to use it sparingly. If you'd rather use another herb instead, marshmallow root is a great replacement.

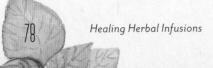

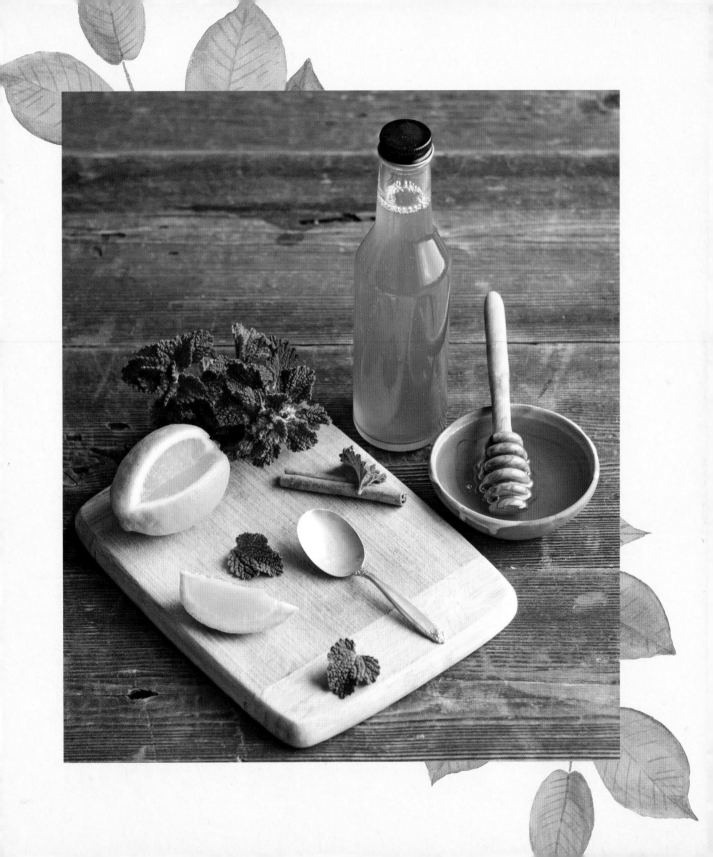

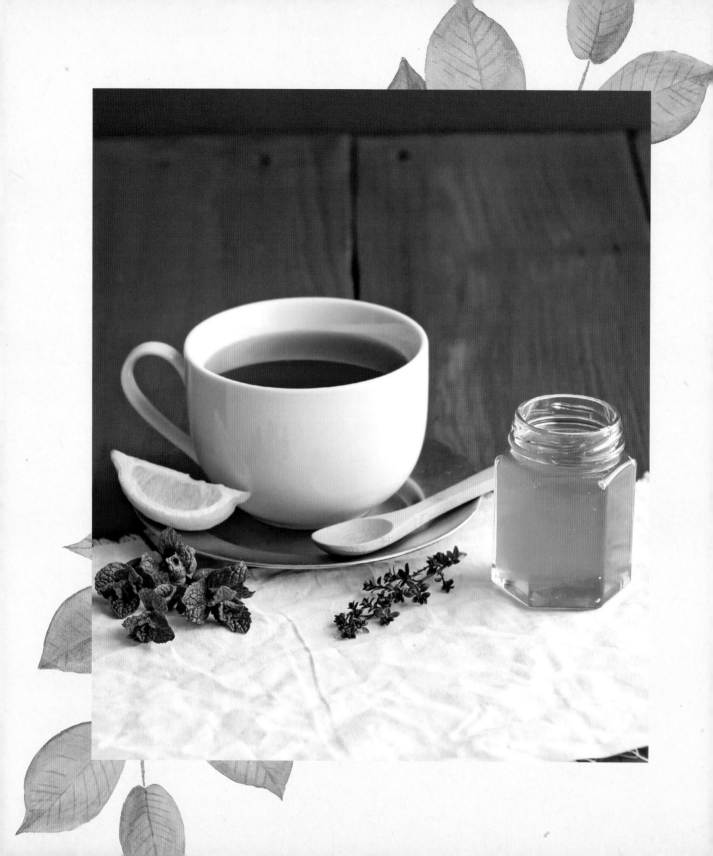

THYME, PEPPERMINT & HONEY TEA FOR COUGHS

Sometimes a handful of herbs from your herb garden is all you need to promote wellness. Thyme and peppermint are especially good for treating persistent coughs, with thyme being a potent natural expectorant and peppermint acting as a decongestant. A few spoonfuls of honey help to coat and soothe the throat, and lemon juice is antibacterial and adds a boost of flavor and vitamin C. Peppermint should be avoided by nursing women as it can reduce your supply. Spearmint is a good alternative with similar benefits.

Yield: about 2 cups (480 ml)

Ingredients
2 cups (480 ml) water

1 tbsp (1 g) fresh thyme

1 tbsp (2 g) fresh or dried peppermint

2–4 tbsp (30–60 ml) raw honey

1 lemon wedge

Instructions
Bring the water to a boil and pour it over the herbs. Let the infusion steep for 10 to 15 minutes, then strain out the herbs and stir in the honey. Add a squeeze of lemon before drinking.

Drink 1 to 2 cups (240 to 480 ml) as often as needed to help relieve and calm a persistent cough.

This tea is safe for children ages 2 and older. Please follow the dosage guidelines on page 23.

Tip: While thyme and peppermint are highly effective for treating coughs, sage, oregano and rosemary are also beneficial and can be substituted if that's what you have growing in your herb garden.

PINE NEEDLE COUGH SYRUP

What better way to make natural medicine than with the trees around us! It turns out that pine needles, along with most other conifer needles, are high in vitamin C and can be used as an expectorant for coughs and for relieving chest congestion. When combined with honey in a syrup, it has the added benefit of being soothing for a dry and scratchy throat and helping to tame the cough. Besides pine, other conifer needles you can use instead are fir, spruce or hemlock (CAUTION: only use the coniferous tree hemlock, not the toxic herbaceous plant also by the same name). Pregnant women should avoid using needles from ponderosa pine.

Yield: about 1½ cups (360 ml)

Ingredients
1¼ cups (300 ml) water

1 cup (16 g) whole, fresh pine needles

½ cup (120 ml) raw honey

Instructions
Bring the water to a boil, then pour it over the pine needles in a pint-size (473-ml) mason jar. Let the infusion steep until the water has cooled to room temperature, then strain out the pine needles and stir in the honey. Store the syrup in a covered jar in the refrigerator and it will keep for 2 to 4 weeks. If you'd like to increase the shelf life of this syrup, freeze it in baggies or ice cube trays and then thaw as needed before use.

Take 1 tablespoon (15 ml) every 2 hours as needed to ease a cough, relieve chest congestion or to soothe a dry and scratchy throat.

This syrup is safe for children ages 2 and older. Please follow the dosage guidelines on page 23.

Tip: Beyond being medicinal, this syrup is very tasty and is nice to have around for the holiday season for mixing into cocktails or mocktails.

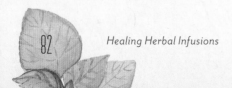

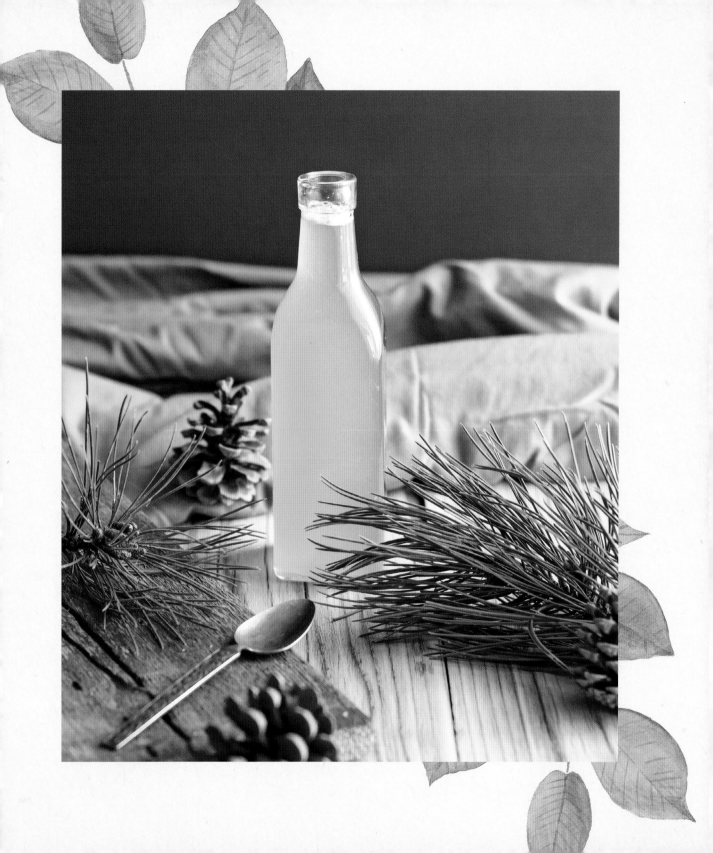

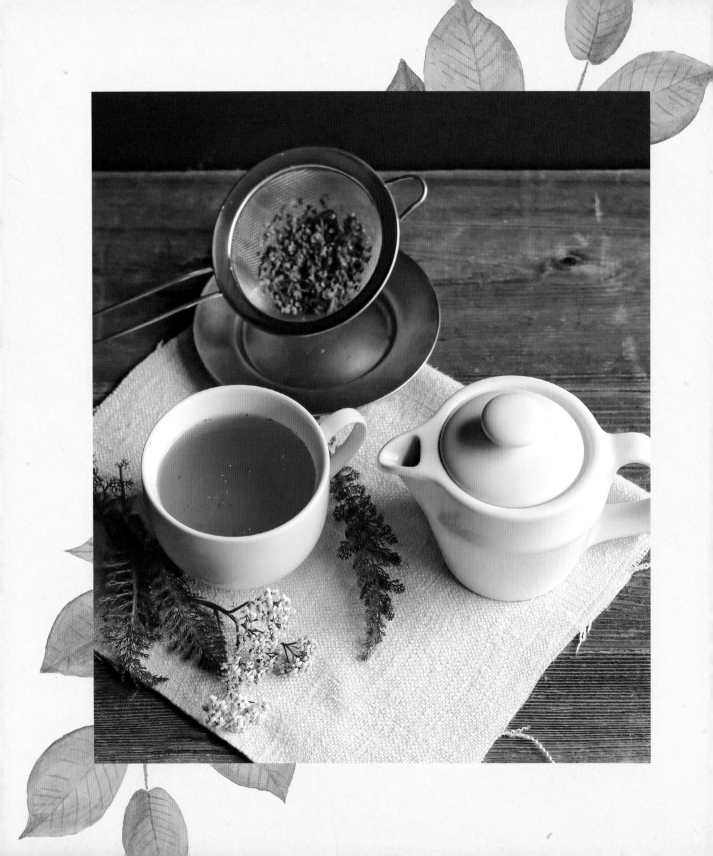

FEVER-REDUCING TEA

Yarrow is arguably one of the best herbs for reducing a fever. It opens up the pores and encourages the body to sweat the fever out, acting as a natural detoxifier. Catnip is relaxing and also encourages sweating. Elderflower also helps to safely bring down a fever, and can be wildcrafted in many areas during the summertime. I always make sure that I harvest and dry some elderflowers each year to have on hand. Cinnamon is warming and offsets the bitter flavor of yarrow. This should always be ingested as a hot tea, so as to promote perspiration. Mild fevers are actually beneficial to the body for fighting infection, but a high fever can become dangerous. If you or someone you are caring for has a high fever, please consult your doctor. Pregnant women should avoid taking yarrow.

Yield: about 2 cups (480 ml)

Ingredients

2 cups (480 ml) water
1 tbsp (3 g) dried yarrow flowers
1 tbsp (1 g) dried catnip
1 tbsp (1 g) dried elderflowers
1 tsp (2 g) cinnamon chips

Instructions

Bring the water to a boil and pour it over the dried herbs. Let the infusion steep for 10 to 15 minutes, then strain out the herbs before drinking.

Drink 1 to 2 cups (240 to 480 ml) piping hot to help sweat out and reduce a fever. If the fever is unusually high, persists for more than a few days or becomes worse, please consult your doctor.

This tea is safe for children ages 2 and older. Please follow the dosage guidelines on page 23. For a milder tasting tea, the yarrow can be omitted.

Tip: These herbs can also be used externally for fevers by infusing them into a hot bath to promote sweating. This is especially helpful for babies and young children.

MULLEIN FLOWER EARACHE OIL

Ear infections are a common ailment of young children, and often antibiotics are the first thing given. The truth of the matter is that not all ear infections need antibiotics to get better, and there is a wonderful herbal alternative that can help to heal and ease the pain of an earache. Mullein flowers are antimicrobial and anti-inflammatory, and they have natural pain-relieving properties. Mullein is an easy to recognize wild plant with its tall yellow flower spike. It grows readily in most areas and is sometimes even considered a noxious weed. Many weeds of this nature have immense benefits to us, and mullein is no exception. Collect and dry the yellow flowers during the summer to have on hand, especially for this earache remedy!

Yield: about ¾ cup (180 ml)

Ingredients
½ cup (8 g) dried mullein flowers
¾ cup (180 ml) olive oil

Instructions
Combine the mullein flowers and the olive oil in a half-pint (236-ml) jar. Cover the jar with a lid and shake to mix well. Put the jar in a cool, dark place to infuse for 4 to 6 weeks. Strain out the herbs with a fine-mesh sieve before using.

When ready to use, warm the oil gently by placing the jar of oil in some warm water. Have the person tilt their head or lay on their side, then use a dropper to place 2 to 3 drops of the warmed oil into the affected ear. Gently massage the outside of the ear for 2 to 3 minutes to facilitate the oil going into the ear canal.

This process can be repeated 3 to 4 times per day to ease earache pain and to eliminate infection. If the pain persists for more than 24 hours, please consult your doctor.

This earache oil is safe to use for children ages 2 and older. For children under the age of 8, only 1 to 2 drops is needed.

Tip: Many recipes for mullein flower oil call for adding fresh garlic, which makes sense given garlic's powerful antibacterial and antimicrobial properties. This concerns me a little, however, because of the potential of botulism, especially in a preparation that will likely be used on children. If you would like to add some garlic to the oil infusion, 1 tablespoon (10 g) of dried garlic granules or pieces (not powdered) is a much safer alternative.

Healing Herbal Infusions

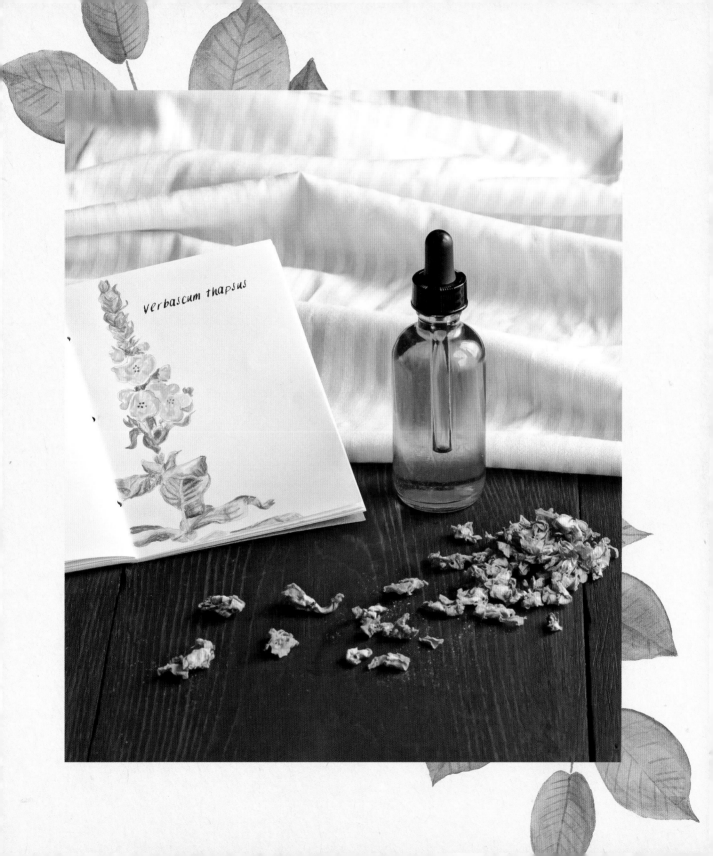

verbascum thapsus

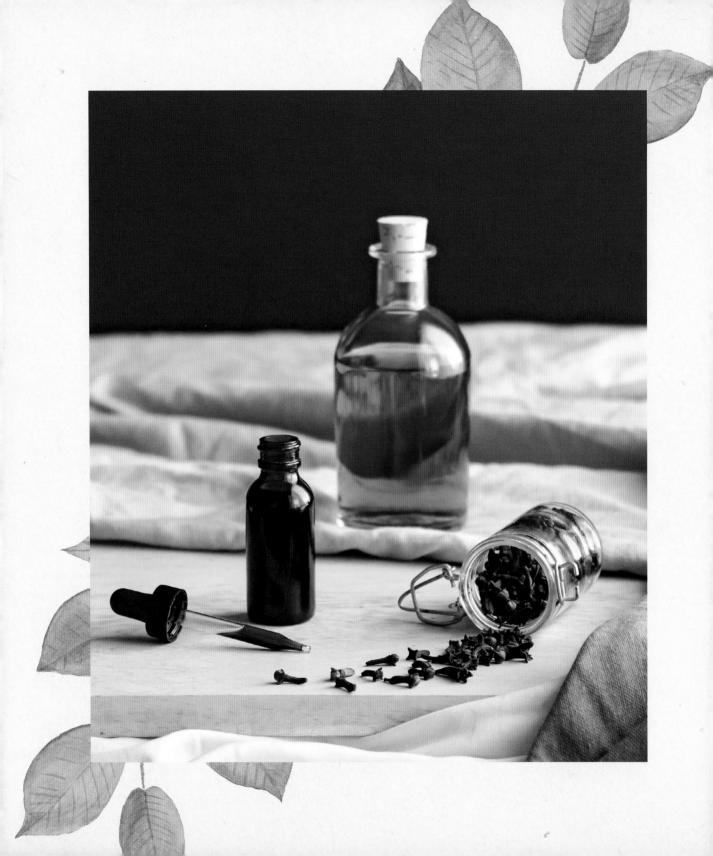

CLOVE WHISKEY TINCTURE FOR TOOTH PAIN

Toothaches can be a real bummer, especially when you can't get in to see the dentist right away. This tincture will help relieve the pain while you're waiting for your appointment. Cloves are well known for numbing tooth pain; it's actually amazing how well they work! Whiskey used topically on teeth can also help to lessen the severity of the pain. If you're prone to having tooth pain, make up this clove tincture to always have on hand. Please note that no more than a few drops at a time should be ingested internally, as large amounts of cloves can be toxic. This tincture should not be used on exposed gums after a tooth extraction or as a remedy for teething babies—it's much too strong for those purposes.

Yield: about ¾ cup (180 ml)

Ingredients
¼ cup (20 g) whole cloves
¾ cup (180 ml) whiskey

Instructions
Combine the cloves and whiskey in a half-pint (236-ml) jar, then cover with a lid. Put in a cool, dark place to infuse for 4 to 6 weeks. Strain out the cloves when ready to use.

Rub the tincture on the affected tooth using your finger or a cotton swab to dull the pain, up to 3 times daily. If the pain persists for more than a day or two, please consult with your dentist.

I do not recommend children under the age of 18 use this tincture. Children over the age of 12 and those wishing to avoid using alcohol can use a drop or two of high-quality clove essential oil to help relieve tooth pain.

Tip: If you would rather not use whiskey in this tincture, feel free to substitute with vodka, brandy or rum.

HAWTHORN & HIBISCUS TEA FOR THE HEART

Both hawthorn berries and hibiscus flowers are known for being beneficial for the heart, which is fitting given their red color. Hawthorn berries are an overall heart tonic used for preventing heart problems as well as helping to treat heart disease by dilating the arteries and veins and releasing blockages. They, along with hibiscus flowers, are also highly efficient at lowering blood pressure, so much so that some people have been able to reduce or even discontinue taking prescription blood pressure medication. If you have heart issues, or are on blood pressure medication, please consult with your doctor first before using this tea. Pregnant women should avoid using hibiscus.

Yield: about 2 cups (480 ml)

Ingredients
2 cups (480 ml) water
1 tbsp (10 g) dried hawthorn berries
2 tbsp (6 g) dried hibiscus flowers

Instructions
Bring the water to a boil and pour it over the dried berries and flowers. Let the infusion steep for 10 to 15 minutes, then strain out the herbs before drinking. For a stronger tea, follow the directions on page 15 for an overnight infusion. This tea can be consumed cold or hot.

Drink daily, as often as needed, to help lower blood pressure and to prevent heart disease.

While children generally do not need the heart effects of this tea, it is still safe for those ages 2 and older. Please follow the dosage guidelines on page 23.

Tip: Fresh hawthorn berries make a wonderful jam, or you can use the dried berries to make jelly. Get some heart-healthy benefits on your morning toast!

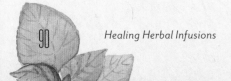

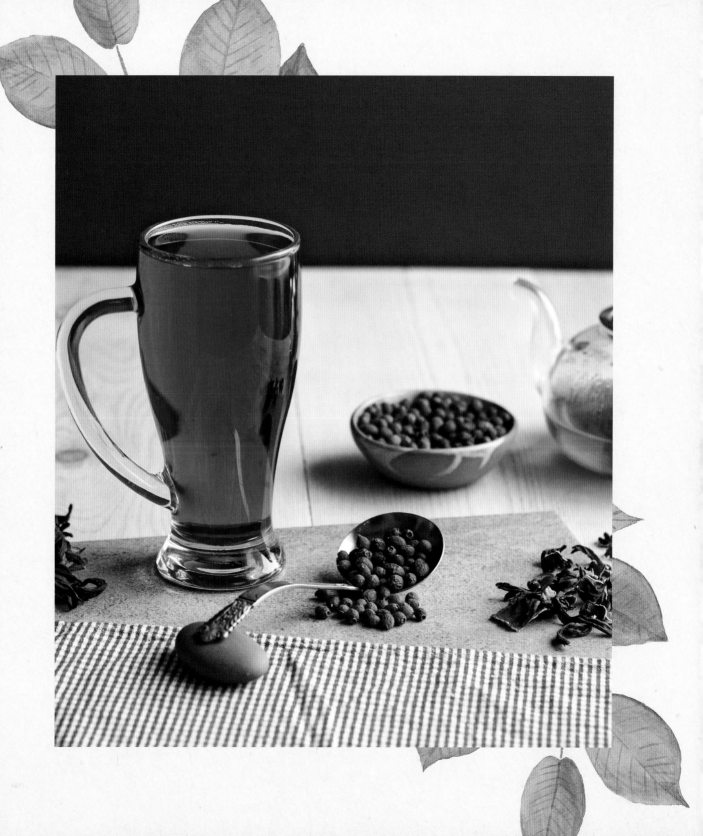

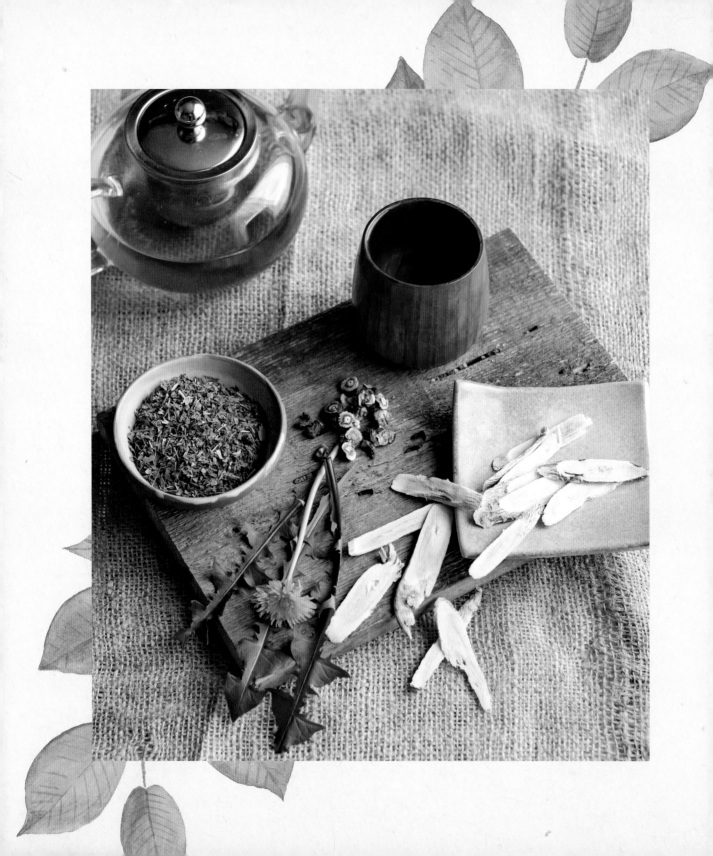

Check Out Receipt

KDL
Kent District Library
www.kdl.org

KDL Plainfield Township Branch

Items that you checked out

Title: Better homes and gardens
ID: 31298029640805
Due: Wednesday, May 29, 2019

Total items: 1
Account balance: $0.00
5/22/2019 1:09 PM
Checked out: 11
Overdue: 0
Hold requests: 15
Ready for pickup: 0

Thank you for using the KDL SelfCheck
System.
Thank you for visiting
KDL Plainfield Township Branch
616 784-2007
www.kdl.org

LIVER SUPPORT TONIC

This is a gentle yet powerful tea infusion that helps to support the health of your liver. Dandelion root is well known as a liver cleanser and detoxifier, and it has a bitter quality that encourages proper digestion. Astragalus root stimulates the liver, and nettles are nourishing for both the liver and kidneys. I admit that this isn't the tastiest infusion, but roasting the dandelion root ahead of time, adding a few dried hibiscus flowers or stirring in a bit of sweetener can make it a little more palatable.

Yield: about 2 cups (480 ml)

Ingredients
2 cups (480 ml) water
1 tbsp (7 g) dandelion root
4–5 slices (4 g) dried astragalus root broken into pieces
1 tbsp (2 g) dried nettles

Instructions
Bring the water to a boil and pour over the dried herbs. Let the infusion steep for 10 to 15 minutes, then strain out the herbs before drinking. For a stronger tea, follow the directions on page 15 for an overnight infusion.

Drink 1 to 2 cups (240 to 480 ml) daily whenever needed for extra liver support.

While children generally do not need the liver-detoxing effects of this tea, it is still safe for those ages 2 and older. Please follow the dosage guidelines on page 23.

Tip: Some other liver-friendly herbs you can use are milk thistle seed, chicory root, burdock root or yellow dock root.

UTI RELIEF TEA

If you've ever had one, then you know that urinary tract infections are no picnic. I used to get them frequently, but this tea saved me! It helps to heal a UTI naturally, and it allows your body to build up the antibodies necessary to effectively fight off any recurrent infections. Since I started using this tea as a remedy, I haven't had a UTI in more than 10 years! Uva ursi, yarrow, dandelion root and juniper berries all have a diuretic effect, which helps to flush the infection out, and marshmallow root is soothing to the urinary tract. Uva ursi, also known as bearberry or kinnikinnick, is astringent and a powerful urinary antiseptic, and it is the most important herb in this remedy (take it if you have nothing else). A couple of things to note about uva ursi: It should not be taken for more than a week at a time, and it is not a suitable herb for children ages 12 and under.

Yield: about 2 cups (480 ml)

Ingredients
2 cups (480 ml) water
1 tbsp (6 g) dried uva ursi
1 tbsp (3 g) dried yarrow
2 tsp (4 g) dried dandelion root
2 tsp (1 g) dried juniper berries
1 tsp (1 g) dried marshmallow root

Instructions
Bring the water to a boil and pour it over the dried herbs. Let the infusion steep for 10 to 15 minutes, then strain out the herbs before drinking.

Drink 1 cup (240 ml) 2 to 3 times per day at the very first sign of a urinary tract infection to help flush it out and promote healing. Do not take for more than 1 week. If symptoms don't show any sign of improvement, or become worse after 24 hours, please consult your doctor.

This tea is safe for children ages 13 and older. Please follow the dosage guidelines on page 23. For use on children under the age of 13, omit the uva ursi and then it is safe for ages 2 and older.

Tip: Vitamin C can actually make a UTI worse, so discontinue any vitamin C supplements you may be taking and hold off on the orange juice. Cranberry juice is still considered an effective UTI remedy, but it absolutely must be the unsweetened variety.

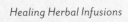

Healing Herbal Infusions

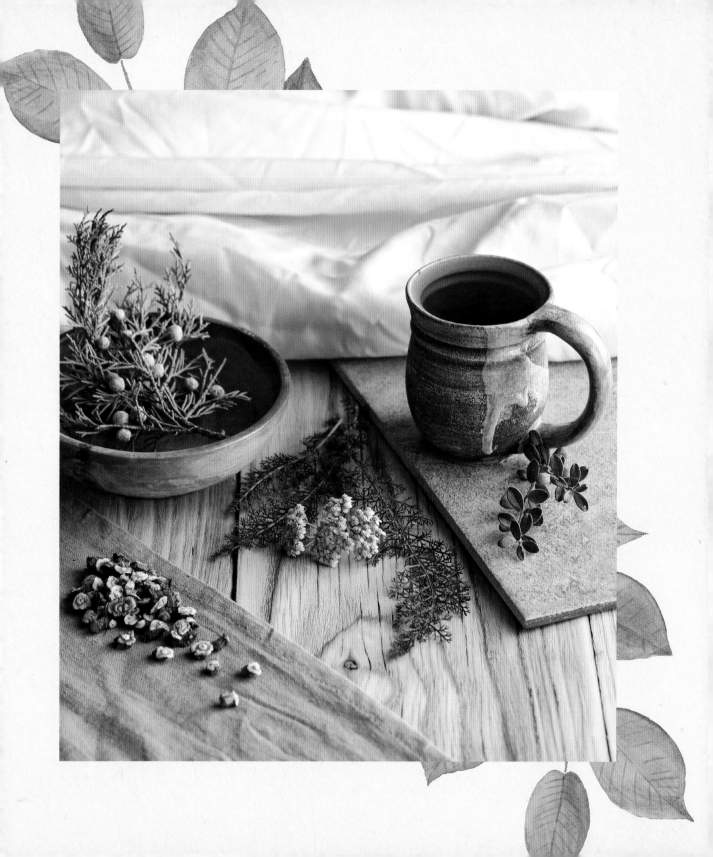

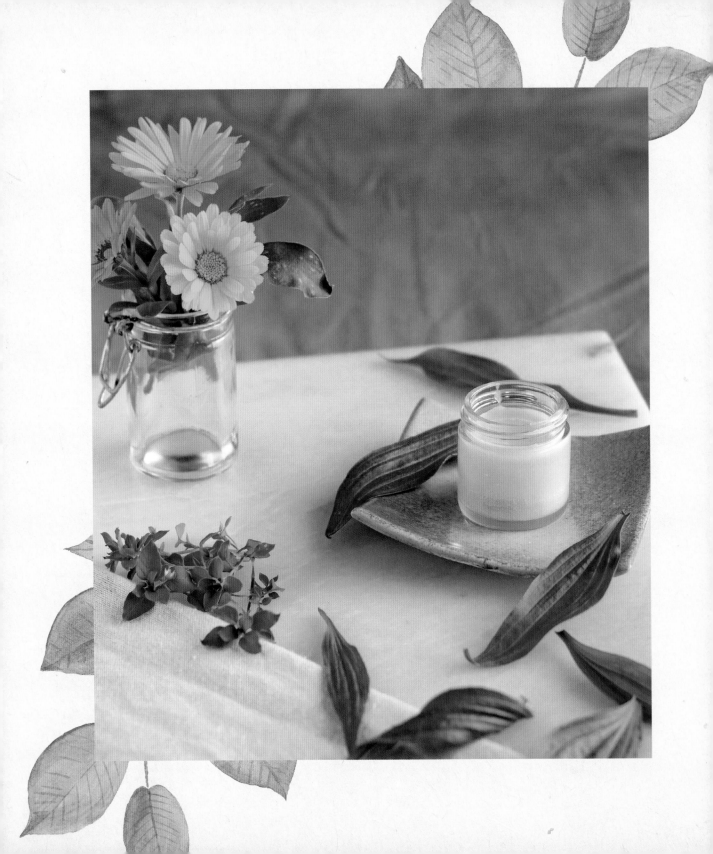

ECZEMA RELIEF SALVE

The itchiness and discomfort caused by eczema can be hard to deal with, but this salve will make it a bit easier! It is made with three herbs that work together to help relieve eczema: calendula flowers speed healing, plantain stops the itch and chickweed is extra moisturizing. Coconut oil is anti-inflammatory, and sweet almond and apricot kernel oils are super hydrating. I use double the amount of shea butter in this salve than what I normally use in my other salves because of its healing effect on eczema. Finally, the natural relief that you've been looking for—and it really works! Note that while this salve is especially good for eczema, it can also be used to help relieve any other dry and itchy skin ailments you may have.

Yield: about 6 ounces (180 ml) of salve

Ingredients

For the Infused Oil

¼ cup (5 g) dried calendula flowers

2 tbsp (5 g) dried plantain leaf

2 tbsp (5 g) dried chickweed

¼ cup (60 ml) coconut oil, melted

¼ cup (60 ml) sweet almond oil

¼ cup (60 ml) apricot kernel oil

For the Salve

½ cup (120 ml) herb-infused oil

½ oz (14 g) beeswax

1 oz (28 g) shea butter

Instructions

Combine the calendula, plantain and chickweed with the coconut, sweet almond and apricot kernel oils in a half-pint (236-ml) jar. Cover the jar with a lid and shake to mix well. Put the jar in a cool, dark place to infuse for 4 to 6 weeks.

When you are ready to make the salve, strain the herbs from the oil using a fine-mesh sieve. If the coconut oil has solidified in the oil infusion, gently heat it by setting the jar in a pan of warm water to melt the oil before straining. Measure out ½ cup (120 ml) of the infused oil, saving any excess oil for later use if you wish. Put the oil into a double boiler on medium heat (see tips for making your own double boiler on page 20). Add the beeswax to the oil and continue to heat until all of the beeswax has completely melted. Next, add the shea butter, and when it has melted, remove the mixture from the heat. Carefully pour the mixture into jars or tins. Let the salve cool and set up for 3 to 4 hours before use.

Apply as often as needed to help heal, relieve the itch and soothe the pain caused by eczema.

This eczema salve is safe to use on children ages 6 months and older following a patch test (see page 23).

LEMON BALM COLD SORE BALM

I absolutely love my patch of lemon balm in the backyard! Lemon balm is a very easy herb to grow or forage for, and can even sometimes become invasive. That is not a problem for me because it has so many healing benefits. It looks similar to mint—it's in the same family—and it has a characteristic lemony scent. One of the greatest things lemon balm can do is help to improve cold sore symptoms and shorten the duration of healing time. Lemon balm is also effective at relieving headache pain (see page 73), reducing stress (see page 185) and keeping mosquitoes away.

Yield: about 6 ounces (180 ml) of lip balm

Ingredients

For the Infused Oil
½ cup (14 g) dried lemon balm

½ cup (120 ml) coconut oil, melted

¼ cup (60 ml) olive oil

1 tbsp (15 ml) castor oil

For the Balm
½ cup (120 ml) herb-infused oil

1 oz (28 g) beeswax

½ oz (14 g) shea butter

10 drops lavender essential oil

Instructions

Combine the lemon balm with the coconut, olive and castor oils in a half-pint (236-ml) jar. Cover the jar with a lid and shake to mix well. Put the jar in a cool, dark place to infuse for 4 to 6 weeks.

When you are ready to make the lip balm, strain the herb from the oil using a fine-mesh sieve. If the coconut oil has solidified in the oil infusion, gently heat it by setting the jar in a pan of warm water to melt the oil before straining. Measure out ½ cup (120 ml) of the infused oil, saving any excess oil for later use if you wish. Put the oil into a double boiler on medium heat (see tips for making your own double boiler on page 20). Add the beeswax to the oil and continue to heat until all of the beeswax has completely melted. Next, add the shea butter, and when it has melted, remove the mixture from the heat. Stir in the lavender essential oil, then carefully pour the mixture into jars, tins or lip balm tubes. Let the lip balm cool and set up for 3 to 4 hours before use.

Apply as often as needed to help improve cold sore symptoms and shorten their duration.

This lip balm is safe to use on children ages 2 years and older following a patch test (see page 23). Omit the lavender essential oil for those under age 13.

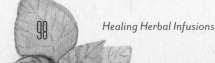

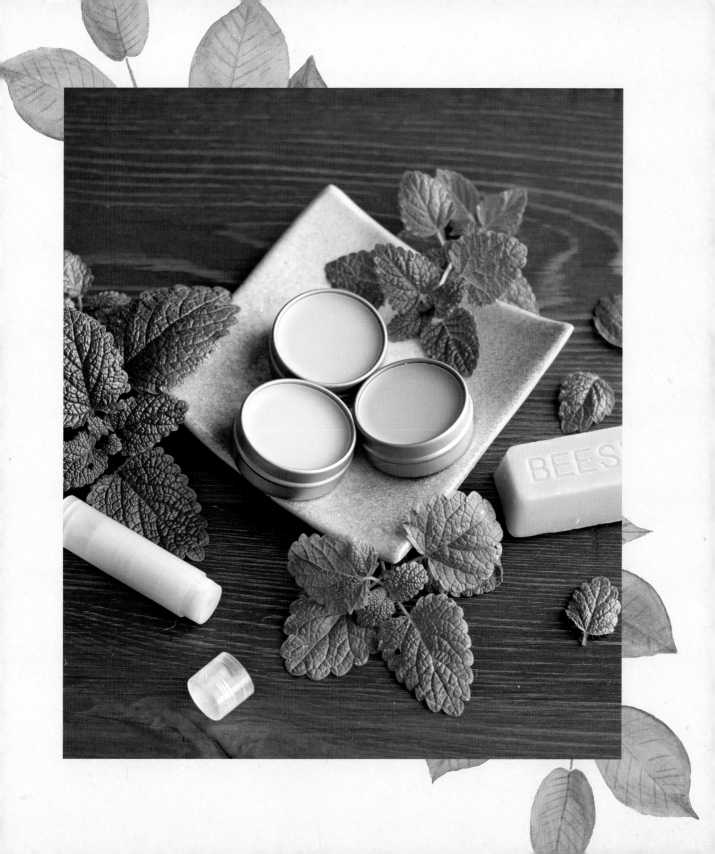

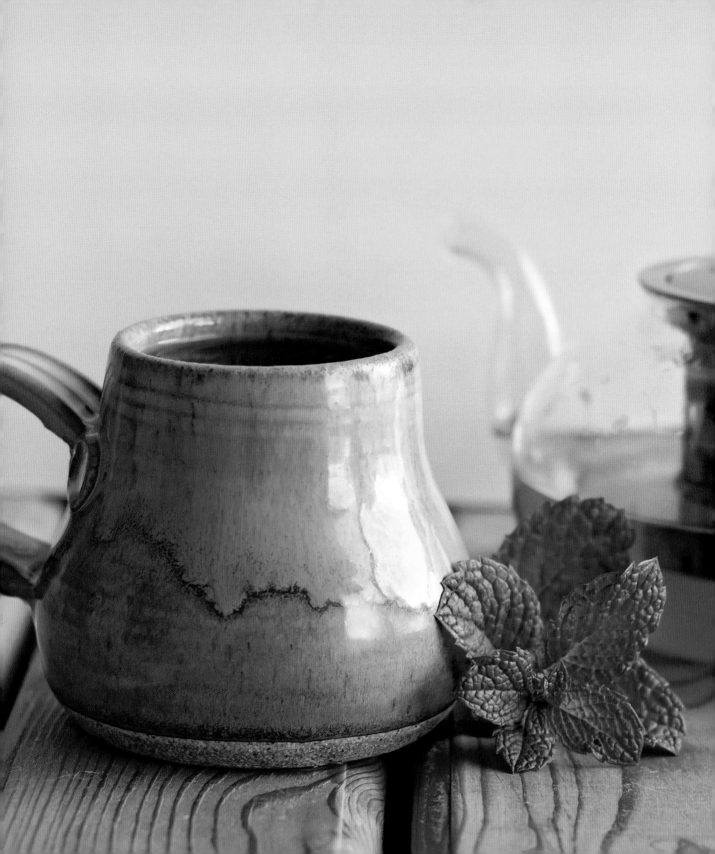

INFUSIONS TO EASE YOUR DIGESTION

Some say that the key to good health starts with the gut. Digestive issues are a very common complaint, from heartburn to upset stomachs. Herbal tea infusions are particularly beneficial for easing digestion, using herbs such as ginger, fennel, cardamom and mint. Bitter herbs such as the roots of dandelion, burdock and chicory are another way of promoting good digestive health, by stimulating the production of bile. Acid reflux can be tamed with a vinegar infusion, and prebiotic herbs can increase the number of probiotics in your gut, keeping everything in check. Reach for these simple infusions before or after a meal to keep your tummy happy and healthy!

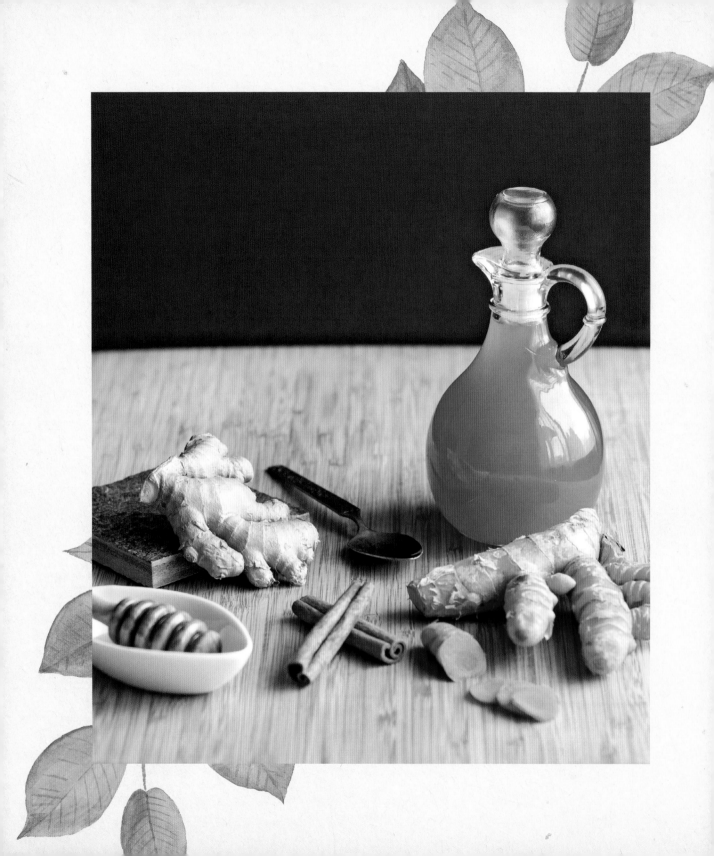

GINGER & TURMERIC DECOCTION & HONEY SYRUP

This is one of my very favorite recipes in this book for two reasons: it has multiple medicinal benefits, and it is also very tasty! When I was pregnant I often had an upset stomach and horrible heartburn. One time I was at a natural foods fair with the worst heartburn I had ever experienced, so I tried a tiny sample of some super potent ginger syrup. My heartburn was immediately gone and stayed away for the rest of the day! I set out to make my own recipe, and this is what I formulated. I use both ginger and turmeric root here because they are both great as a digestive aid, but it is fine to use only ginger if that's all you have access to. Ginger is particularly good for relieving nausea; stir a spoonful of this syrup into sparkling water and you have an instant ginger ale!

Yield: about 2 cups (480 ml)

Ingredients
½ cup (50 g) sliced fresh ginger
½ cup (50 g) sliced fresh turmeric
1 cinnamon stick
2 cups (480 ml) water
½–1 cup (120–240 ml) raw honey

Instructions
Combine the ginger, turmeric, cinnamon stick and water in a small saucepan. Bring to a boil. Reduce the heat slightly and let simmer uncovered for about 20 minutes, or until the liquid has reduced by half. Remove the pan from the heat and let cool to room temperature. Strain out the herbs, then stir in the honey. Start with ½ cup (120 ml) of honey, then add more to taste as needed. Store the syrup in a covered jar in the refrigerator, and it will keep for 2 to 4 weeks. If you'd like to increase the shelf life of this syrup, freeze it in baggies or ice cube trays and then thaw as needed before use. Be forewarned that fresh turmeric can stain and may be hard to remove.

Take 1 tablespoon (15 ml) as needed to help relieve acid reflux/heartburn or an upset stomach. If you prefer, it may also be stirred into a cup of water, sparkling water or tea.

This tea is safe for children ages 2 and older. Please follow the dosage guidelines on page 23. For younger children, it is recommended to dilute in water or tea.

Tip: This syrup is also a powerful immune system booster. Take a spoonful daily to prevent sickness during cold and flu season.

PREBIOTIC HONEY ELECTUARY

An electuary is an old-fashioned type of herbal medicine that is simply herbs, usually in powdered form but not always, combined with honey and used as medicine. This is the perfect way to get more prebiotic herbs into our diet, as the honey helps these herbs go down a bit easier with its sweet taste.

Most everyone knows how good probiotics are for our digestion, but prebiotics are just as important, if not more so. Prebiotics are the food for probiotics, so ingesting them is a great way to naturally increase the probiotics that are already in your gut. Chicory root is especially high in inulin, which is a powerful prebiotic, and dandelion and burdock roots aren't too far behind in inulin content. Marshmallow root also has some prebiotic action, as well as being soothing to the stomach lining. Try using roasted dandelion and chicory root powders for a more pleasing, almost coffee-like flavor.

Yield: about ¾ cup (180 ml)

Ingredients
½ cup (120 ml) raw honey
1 tbsp (6 g) powdered chicory root
1 tbsp (6 g) powdered dandelion root
1 tbsp (6 g) powdered burdock root
1 tbsp (4 g) powdered marshmallow root

Instructions
Combine the honey and powdered roots in a bowl and stir to mix well. Transfer the mixture to a half-pint (236-ml) jar with a lid and store in a cool, dark place. This electuary can be taken immediately or left to infuse for as long as desired before using.

Take 1 tablespoon (15 ml) daily as needed to improve digestion and to promote beneficial bacteria in the gut.

This electuary is safe for children ages 8 and older. Please follow the dosage guidelines on page 23.

Tip: Herbal electuaries aren't used as often as they once were, but they are a highly effective way to ingest powdered herbs in a tasty way. The amounts listed in this recipe are a guideline; feel free to increase the amount of powdered herbs if you'd like. The paste will become thicker, and if you add enough, you will be able to roll little herbal electuary "pills" between your fingers that can be swallowed whole.

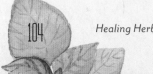

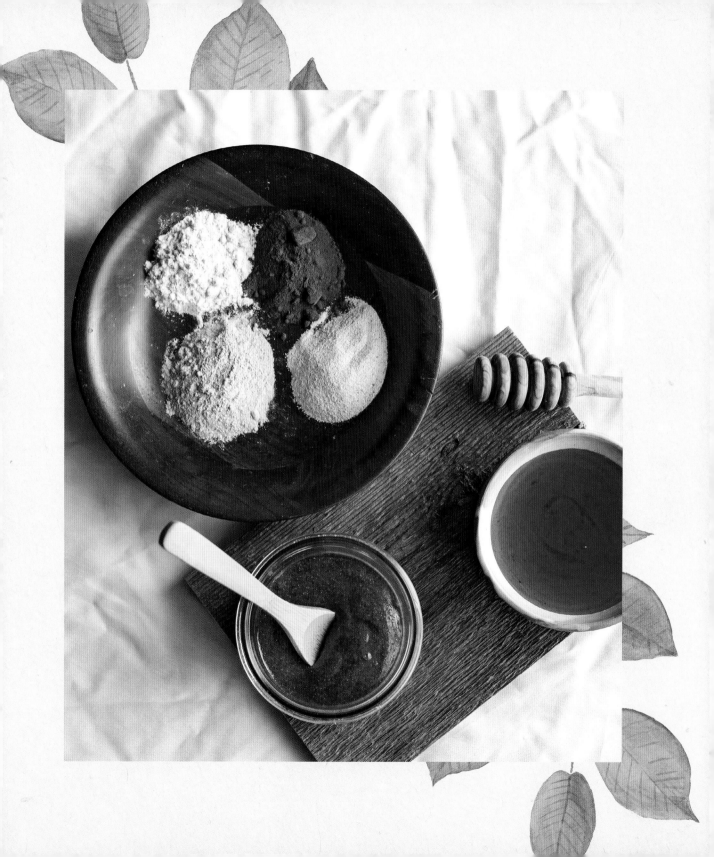

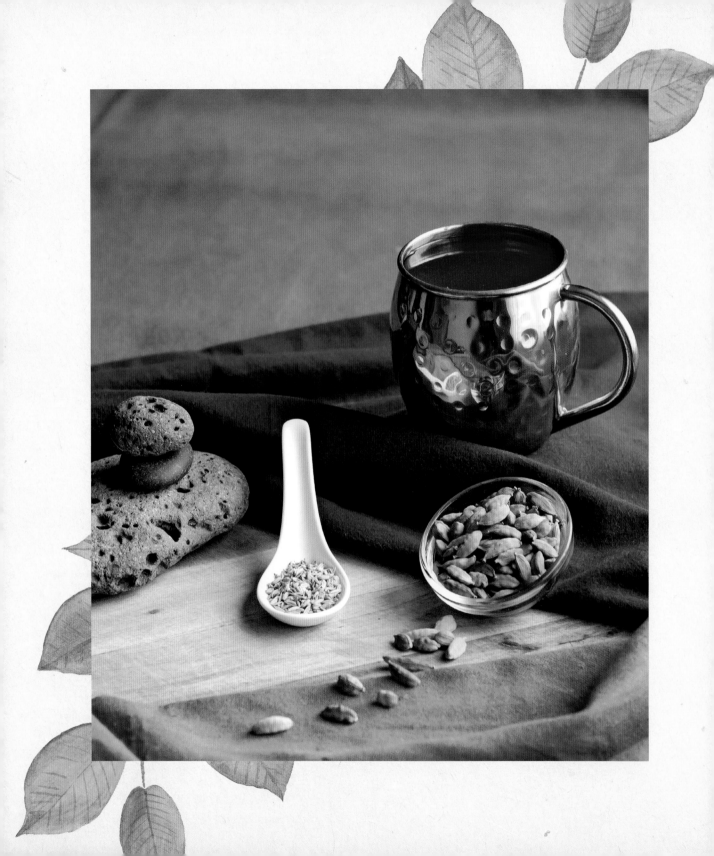

FENNEL & CARDAMOM AFTER-MEAL TUMMY TEA

If you've ever eaten at an Indian food restaurant, you may have noticed a small bowl of fennel seeds, sometimes candy-coated, that are meant to be taken after a meal. This is because fennel seeds are highly effective as a digestive aid and antacid, making them the perfect thing to ingest after a big meal. Cardamom is in the same family as ginger, another digestive superstar. It helps to soothe the stomach and intestines, and it makes food easier to digest. This tea is reminiscent of traditional chai and is a wonderful after-meal drink.

Yield: about 2 cups (480 ml)

Ingredients
1 tbsp (8 g) fennel seed
2 tbsp (20 g) cardamom pods
2½ cups (600 ml) water

Instructions
Combine the fennel, cardamom and water in a small saucepan. Bring to a boil. Reduce the heat to medium-high and simmer for 5 to 10 minutes, then strain out the herbs before drinking.

Drink 1 to 2 cups (240 to 480 ml) after meals to help ease digestion or to soothe an upset stomach.

This tea is safe for children ages 2 and older. Please follow the dosage guidelines on page 23.

Tip: If you need quick digestive help, chew on a ½ teaspoon of whole fennel seeds after a meal for instant relief.

MARSHMALLOW & CINNAMON DIGESTIVE TEA

This soothing digestive tea has marshmallow root as its base, not to be confused with the sugar-laden marshmallows at the grocery store. While traditional marshmallow candy was made with powdered marshmallow root, somehow the version that is popular today has strayed far from its origins. This is unfortunate because eating a piece of real marshmallow candy would be beneficial to the digestive system due to its mucilaginous, stomach-coating effects. This tea works just as well, and a bit of cinnamon makes it tasty while also providing some digestive benefits.

Yield: about 2 cups (480 ml)

Ingredients
2 cups (480 ml) water

2 tbsp (8 g) marshmallow root

2 tsp (5 g) cinnamon chips or ½ cinnamon stick broken into pieces

---

Instructions
Bring the water to a boil and pour it over the dried herbs. Let the infusion steep for 10 to 15 minutes, then strain out the herbs before drinking. This can also be made as a cold-water infusion; see instructions on page 15.

Drink 1 to 2 cups (240 to 480 ml) as often as needed to soothe and repair the digestive system.

This tea is safe for children ages 2 and older. Please follow the dosage guidelines on page 23.

 Tip: Marshmallow plants are easy to grow and are great to have in your medicinal herb garden. They are tall plants in the same family as hollyhocks with pretty white flowers that have a pink center. The one main requirement they have is that they prefer the soil to be consistently wet and "marshy," which is where it gets its name.

Healing Herbal Infusions

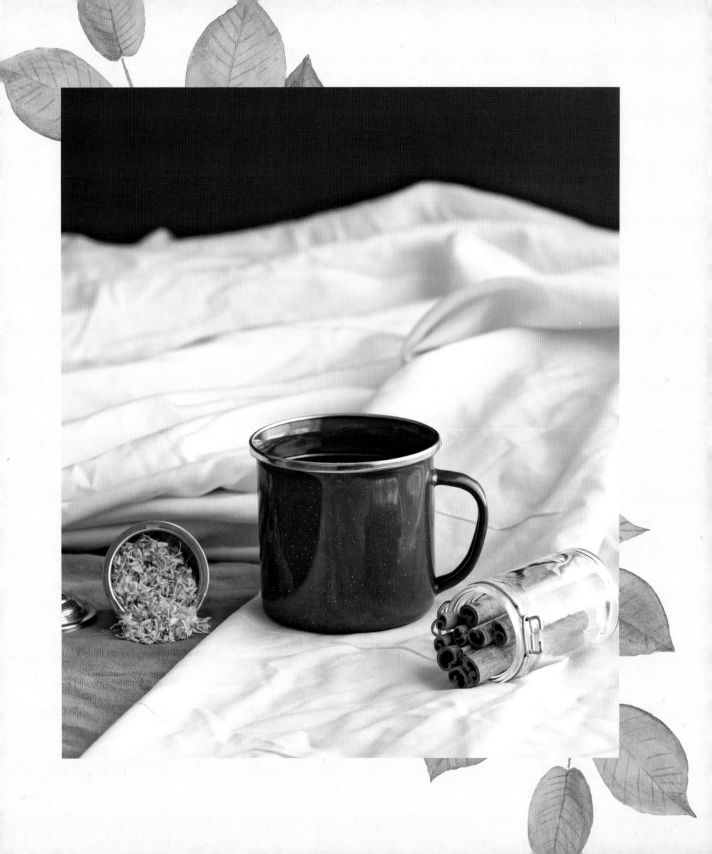

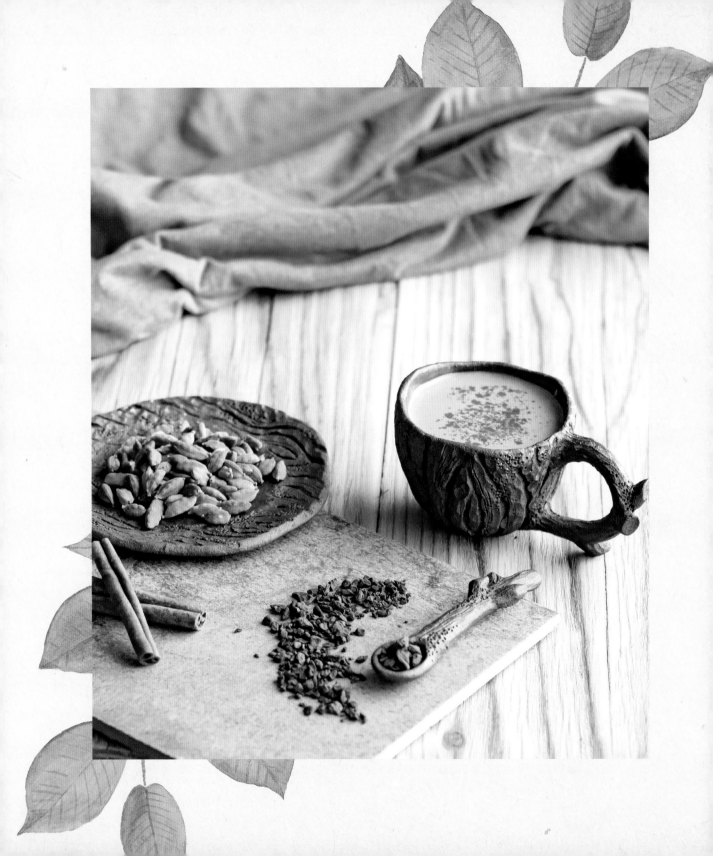

ROASTED CHICORY ROOT CHAI

Chai tea is not generally thought of as a digestive aid, but the main herbs and spices that are used—cardamom, ginger and cinnamon—all have huge benefits for the digestive system. Add in some roasted chicory root, and you have a super gut-healthy and tasty beverage. Chicory root is a prebiotic, meaning that it feeds the beneficial bacteria in the gut microbiome, creating a happy digestive system. The roasted root is rich in flavor and pairs nicely with traditional chai spices.

The beautiful mug in the photo for this recipe was handcrafted by The Wondersmith.

Yield: about 2 cups (480 ml)

Ingredients
2 tbsp (20 g) cardamom pods

1 tbsp (10 g) roasted chicory root

1 tsp (3 g) diced fresh ginger

1 tsp (2 g) dried orange peel

¼ tsp peppercorns

¼ tsp whole cloves

1 cinnamon stick

2½ cups (600 ml) water

Cream or milk

Sweetener, to taste

Instructions
Combine the cardamom, chicory root, ginger, orange peel, peppercorns, cloves, cinnamon stick and water in a small saucepan. Bring to a boil. Reduce the heat to medium-high and simmer for 5 to 10 minutes, then strain out the herbs before drinking. Add cream or milk to make it a traditional chai and a bit of sweetener if you'd like.

Drink 1 to 2 cups (240 to 480 ml) as often as you like to promote healthy digestion.

This tea is safe for children ages 8 and older. Please follow the dosage guidelines on page 23.

Tip: Roasted chicory root also makes a great substitute for coffee when paired with roasted dandelion root. Simply boil 1 tablespoon (10 g) of each dried root for 5 to 10 minutes, then strain and serve.

FOUR-MINTS HERBAL HOT OR ICED TEA

The mint family of herbs is a big one, and many of them have been used throughout history as a digestive aid. Mint is soothing for the stomach and helps with indigestion when consumed after a meal. It is also beneficial to drink before a meal, as it stimulates the flow of bile and digestive enzymes. It also has the added benefit of freshening the breath! Mint leaves are full of volatile oils that give off a wonderful aroma, so I recommend using fresh whenever possible, but dried will work in a pinch.

Yield: about 4 cups (1 L)

Ingredients
4 cups (1 L) water
½ cup (6 g) fresh or 1 tbsp (3 g) dried peppermint leaves
½ cup (6 g) fresh or 1 tbsp (3 g) dried spearmint leaves
½ cup (6 g) fresh or 1 tbsp (2 g) dried lemon balm leaves
½ cup (6 g) fresh or 1 tbsp (1 g) dried catnip leaves

Instructions
Bring the water to a boil and pour it over the herbs in a quart-size (946-ml) mason jar. For a hot tea, let the infusion steep for 15 to 20 minutes, then strain and drink. For an iced tea, let the infusion cool to room temperature, then strain and pour over ice before drinking.

Drink 1 to 2 cups (240 to 480 ml) as often as you like to soothe the stomach and to promote healthy digestion.

This tea is safe for children ages 2 and older. Please follow the dosage guidelines on page 23.

Tip: Other mint-family herbs that work well in this tea are bee balm, lemon bee balm, hyssop, bergamot and purple dead nettle.

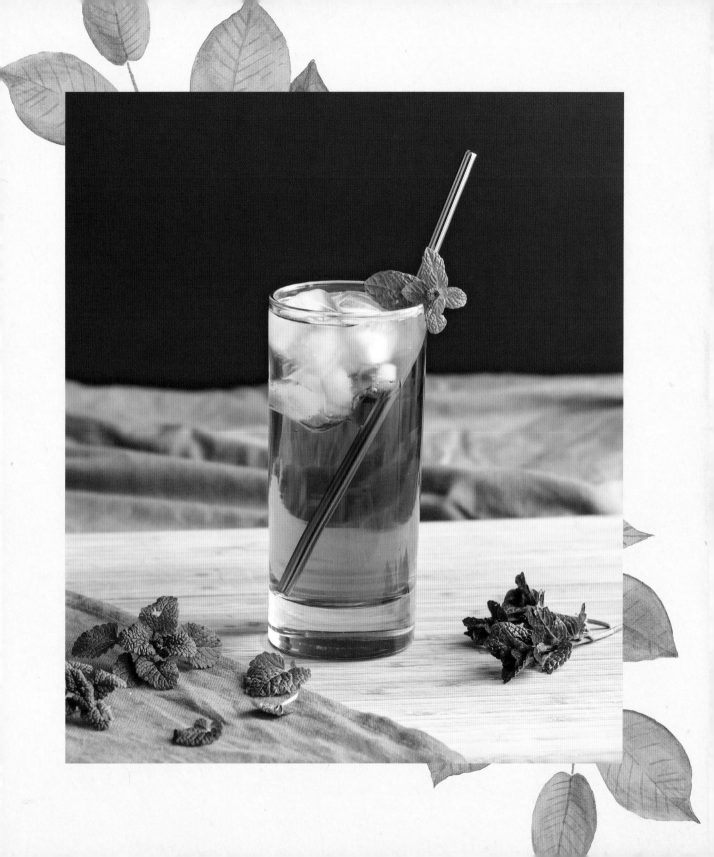

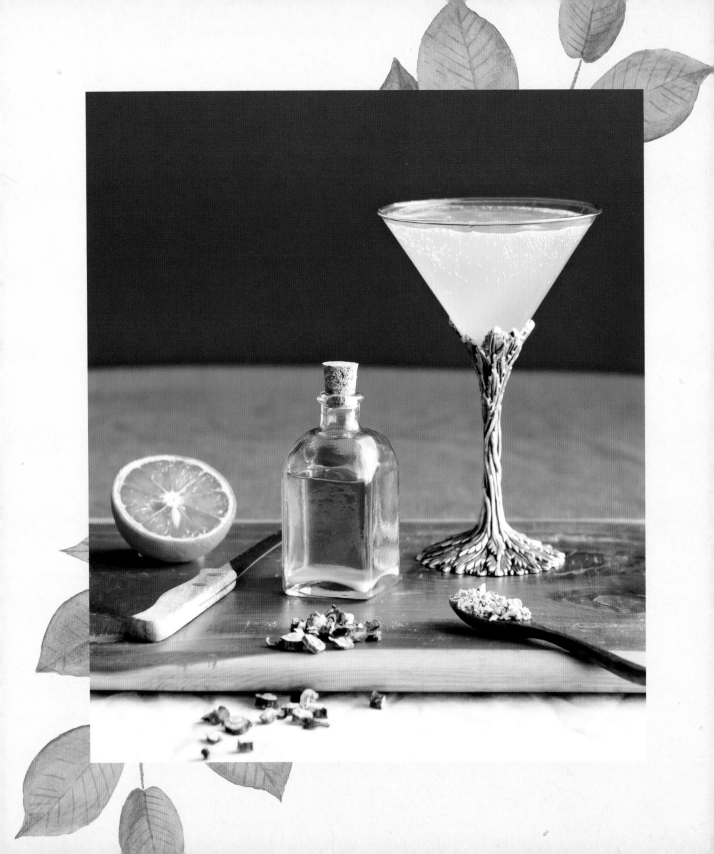

DANDELION & BURDOCK ROOT BITTERS

Bitters are made in the same manner as a tincture, but with bitter herbs as the plant material. Digestive bitters can be sipped straight, mixed with sparkling water or ginger ale or turned into a fancy cocktail to drink before or after a meal. Dandelion and burdock root are bitter herbs that are often paired together, and they are both excellent for digestion. They help to increase and stimulate digestive enzymes and bile production, which both aids digestion and increases the assimilation of nutrients.

Yield: about 1½ cups (360 ml)

Ingredients
2 tbsp (20 g) dried dandelion root

2 tbsp (24 g) dried burdock root

1 tbsp (8 g) dried sweet orange peel

1½ cups (360 ml) vodka or other neutral spirits

Instructions
Combine the herbs and spirits in a pint-size (473-ml) jar. Cover the jar with a lid and shake to mix well. Put the jar in a cool, dark place to infuse for 4 to 6 weeks. Strain out the herbs using a fine-mesh sieve.

Drink up to 1 fluid ounce (30 ml) before or after a meal to help aid digestion or to calm an upset stomach.

Bitters are not meant to be consumed by anyone under the legal drinking age.

Tip: This is pleasantly bitter, and the addition of the orange peel makes it perfect for turning into an aperitif cocktail. Combine it with sparkling water and a splash of orange or grapefruit juice for a lovely drink before a meal.

SARSAPARILLA & FENNEL BITTERS

These bitters have a root beer–like flavor from the sarsaparilla root with a faint anise undertone from the fennel seeds. Sarsaparilla root is one of the traditional flavorings for real old-fashioned root beer, and it has a bitter quality to it. Fennel seeds are highly beneficial for aiding digestion, especially after a meal. Sip straight up or mix into a cocktail for the perfect post-meal drink!

Yield: about 1½ cups (360 ml)

Ingredients
2 tbsp (12 g) dried sarsaparilla root
2 tbsp (18 g) dried fennel seed
1 tbsp (8 g) cinnamon chips
1½ cups (360 ml) vodka or other neutral spirits

Instructions
Combine the herbs and spirits in a pint-size (473-ml) jar. Cover the jar with a lid and shake to mix well. Put the jar in a cool, dark place to infuse for 4 to 6 weeks. Strain out the herbs using a fine-mesh sieve.

Drink up to 1 fluid ounce (30 ml) before or after a meal to help aid digestion or to calm an upset stomach.

Bitters are not meant to be consumed by anyone under the legal drinking age.

Tip: The addition of fennel and cinnamon makes this a great choice for mixing into a digestif cocktail. Combine it with a natural ginger ale (see page 103) and a squeeze of lemon to help digest after a meal.

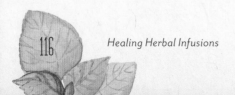

Healing Herbal Infusions

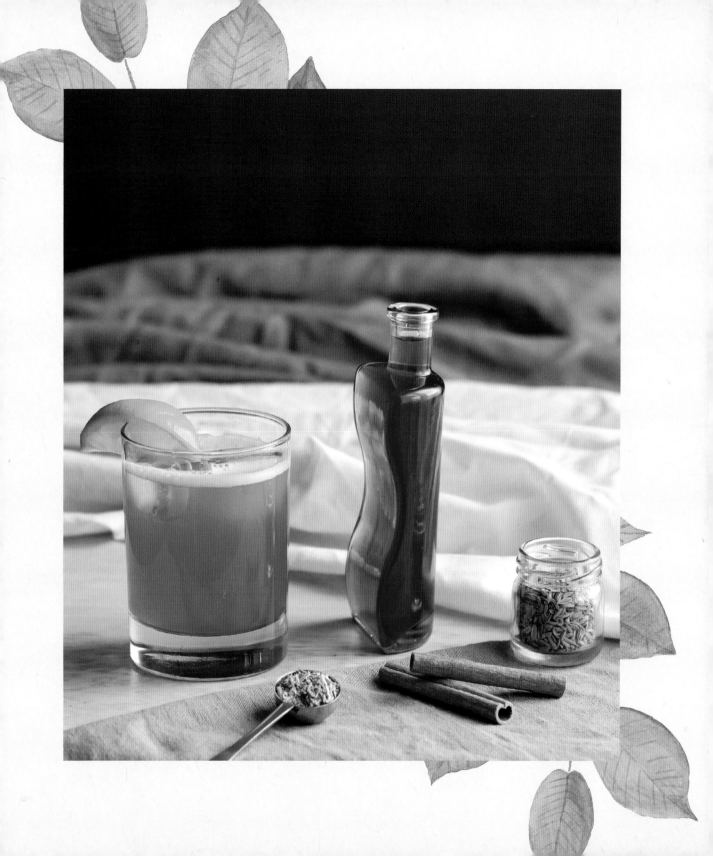

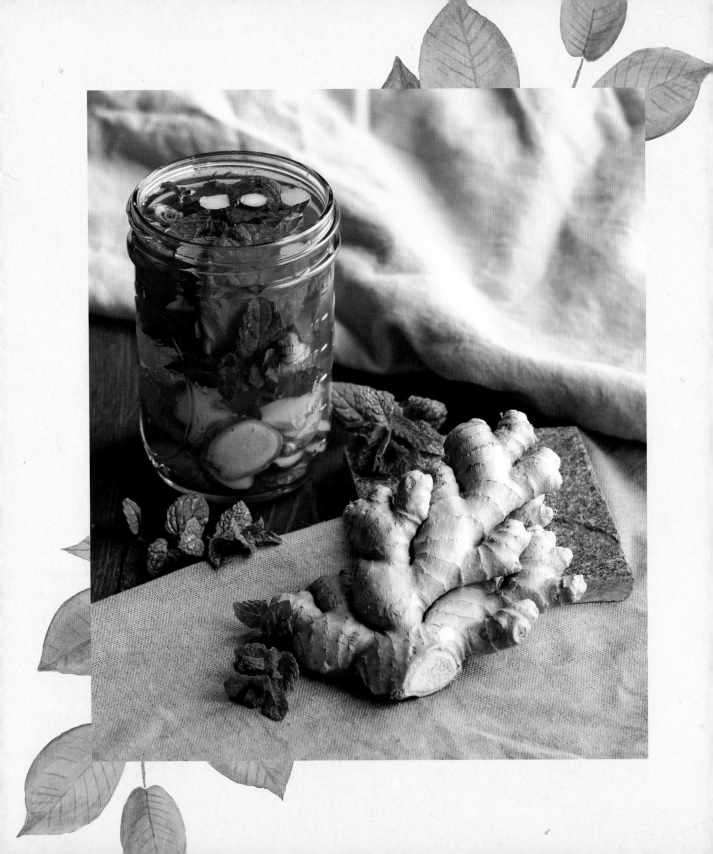

HERBAL VINEGAR INFUSION FOR HEARTBURN

It may seem counterintuitive, but vinegar, particularly raw apple cider vinegar, often provides almost instant relief for acid reflux, more commonly known as heartburn. One theory of why this folk remedy works so well is that heartburn may actually be caused by too little acid in the stomach, and apple cider vinegar helps to neutralize the pH in your gut. The addition of ginger and peppermint, which are both helpful for heartburn as well, makes this infusion even more potent. Honey is a nice addition to improve the flavor if desired, and it can help reduce heartburn as well.

Yield: about 1½ cups (360 ml)

Ingredients
1½ cups (360 ml) raw apple cider vinegar
½ cup (50 g) sliced fresh ginger
½ cup (8 g) loosely packed fresh peppermint leaves
1–3 tbsp (15–45 ml) raw honey (optional)

Instructions
Combine the apple cider vinegar, ginger and peppermint in a pint-size (473-ml) jar. Cover the jar with a lid and put in a cool, dark place to infuse for 4 to 6 weeks. Strain out the herbs when ready to use, then stir in the honey (if using).

Stir 1 tablespoon (15 ml) of the vinegar infusion into a cup of water and drink it as needed to help relieve acid reflux, no more than 3 times daily. If the acid reflux persists for more than a day or two, please consult your doctor.

This vinegar infusion is safe for children ages 2 and older. Please follow the dosage guidelines on page 23 and dilute it with water before using.

Tip: If you don't have this infusion already made, you can simply use 1 tablespoon (15 ml) of plain raw apple cider vinegar diluted in water for quick heartburn relief!

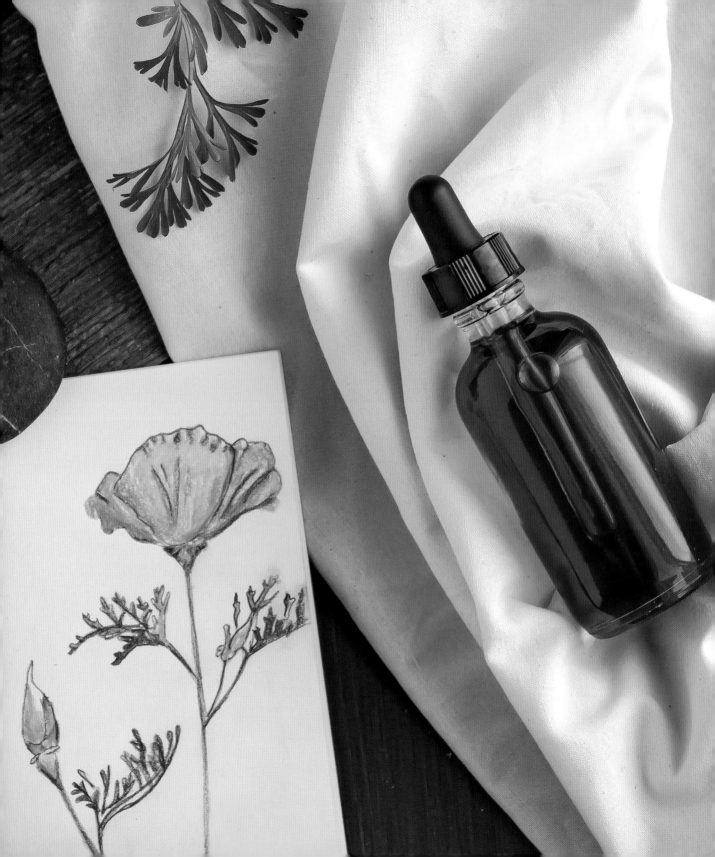

INFUSIONS TO EMBRACE YOUR INNER WELL-BEING

The mind-body connection is an important one. There are many herbs that have mood-enhancing and relaxing properties that can help us in the journey of life. Saint John's wort and California poppy can lift up our emotions and put us in a better state of mind. Valerian, chamomile, catnip, lavender, lemon balm and passionflower have a calming effect and are great for unwinding at the end of a long and stressful day. Holy basil (also known as tulsi) is special in that it can help to maintain the balance of your energy centers, also called "chakras." Nettle and oatstraw can help to replenish vital nutrients that keep us feeling strong. Infused teas, tinctures and massage oils can help us to revitalize, loosen up, calm down and bring on sleep in a natural way—all the while putting a positive herbal energy into our psyche!

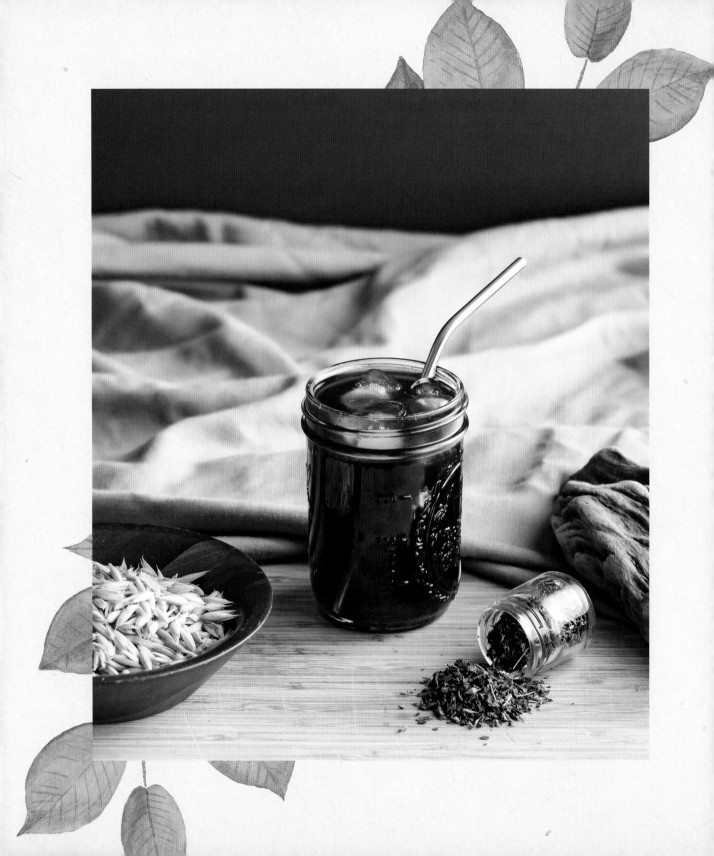

NETTLE & OATSTRAW LONG-INFUSED TEA FOR VITALITY

When you are lacking energy and you need to replenish essential vitamins and minerals, this is the drink to turn to. Stinging nettle is a vitamin- and mineral-rich weed that grows nearly everywhere, and when turned into an infusion, it's like nature's energy drink. Oatstraw is rich in minerals such as calcium and magnesium, and is also high in vitamins and many other trace nutrients. Oatstraw is also effective for treating anxiety and stress. You can use oat tops in place of oatstraw if you prefer; they have a bit of a stronger effect. I particularly like to drink this infusion with a tablespoon (15 ml) of blackstrap molasses stirred in. It improves the flavor while also providing even more minerals!

Yield: about 4 cups (1 L)

Ingredients
4 cups (1 L) water
½ cup (16 g) dried nettles
½ cup (20 g) dried oatstraw or oat tops
1 tbsp (15 ml) honey, maple syrup or blackstrap molasses (optional)

Instructions
Bring the water to a boil and pour it over the herbs in a quart-size (946-ml) mason jar. Cover the jar with a lid and let the infusion steep for 4 to 12 hours. Strain with a fine-mesh sieve and add the sweetener, if you'd like, before drinking. This infusion is best when consumed cold over ice.

Drink 1 to 4 cups (240ml to 1 L) daily to replenish nutrients and to revitalize the mind and body.

This tea is safe for children ages 2 and older. Please follow the dosage guidelines on page 23.

Tip: Fresh stinging nettles can be used instead of dried if you have access to them. Use enough to fill your quart (946-ml) jar about half full with fresh nettles, and be sure to use a fine-mesh sieve lined with a few layers of cheesecloth to remove all of the fine hairs before drinking. Be careful of their sting when harvesting nettles—wearing gloves is recommended. No need to worry about the sting in the finished infusion, the boiling water will completely deaden it.

SLEEP WELL TEA

Sometimes sleep can elude us, but there are herbs that can help us enter into the dream world peacefully. Chamomile, a gentle herb that promotes restfulness and reduces stress, is one that you may have heard of and might already have in your tea cupboard. Catnip isn't just for your feline friends, but is soothing to the nervous system and helps to relieve pain. Valerian is a powerful herb that is commonly used for sleeplessness, as it is calming for jittery nerves and beneficial for treating insomnia. One mug full of this infusion and you should be drifting to sleep in no time!

Yield: about 2 cups (480 ml)

Ingredients
2 cups (480 ml) water
1 tbsp (1 g) dried chamomile flowers
1 tbsp (2 g) dried catnip
1 tsp (2 g) dried valerian root

Instructions
Bring the water to a boil and pour it over the dried herbs. Let the infusion steep for 10 to 15 minutes, then strain out the herbs before drinking. For a stronger tea, follow the directions on page 15 for a long or overnight infusion.

Drink 1 to 2 cups (240 to 480 ml) before bedtime to help relax and to promote restful sleep.

This tea is safe for children ages 2 and older. Please follow the dosage guidelines on page 23. For a milder tea for sleep and relaxation, try Children's Calming Tea on page 185.

Tip: Valerian root is helpful for treating chronic insomnia, but it may take a few weeks for the effects to be noticeable. Drink this tea every night for 2 weeks and you may notice sleep finding you more easily than before. It is also advised to take a week off from taking valerian root every 2 to 3 weeks.

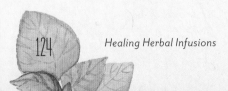

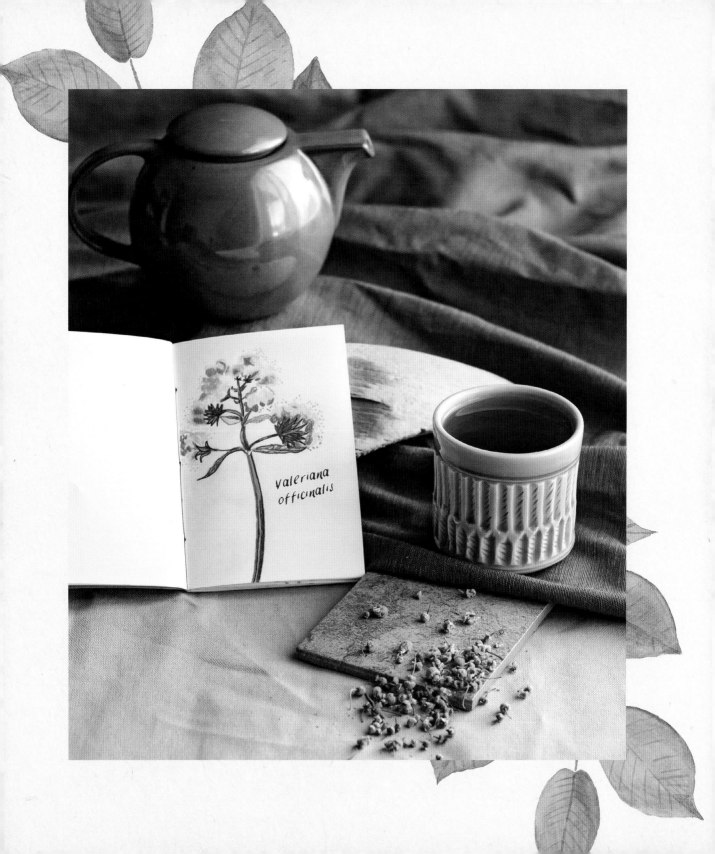

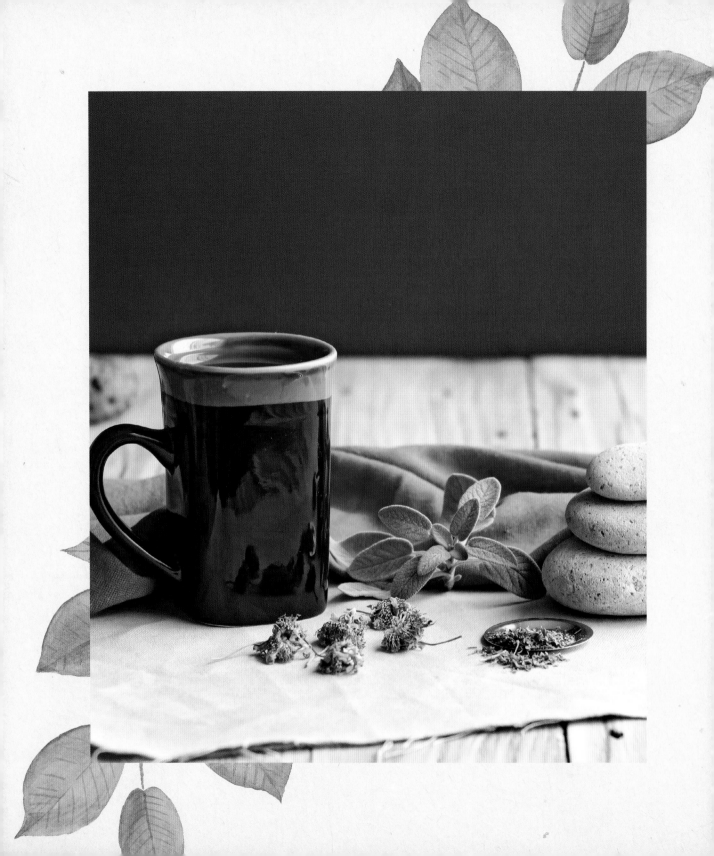

DE-STRESS TEA

Emotional stress is unfortunately something that we all deal with from time to time, but there are herbs that can help. Holy basil is particularly good at this, being an adaptogenic herb that relieves stress and anxiety, reduces cortisol and promotes relaxation. Passionflower lowers blood pressure, reduces depression and improves sleep. Sage helps to tame frazzled nerves. This is a flavorful tea that even has a calming aromatherapy effect when inhaled. Pregnant women should avoid using large amounts of holy basil and passionflowers.

Yield: about 2 cups (480 ml)

Ingredients
2 cups (480 ml) water
2 tbsp (3 g) dried or ¼ cup (6 g) fresh holy basil (tulsi)
1 tbsp (3 g) dried or ¼ cup (6 g) fresh passionflowers
5–6 (2 g) fresh sage leaves

Instructions
Bring the water to a boil and pour it over the herbs. Let the infusion steep for 10 to 15 minutes, then strain out the herbs before drinking. For a stronger tea, follow the directions on page 15 for a long or overnight infusion. This tea can be consumed hot or iced.

Drink 1 to 2 cups (240 to 480 ml) daily as needed to help reduce stress and anxiety.

This tea is safe for children ages 2 and older. Please follow the dosage guidelines on page 23.

Tip: Holy basil, also known as tulsi, is truly an amazing herb. It helps to restore vitality, renews energy and balances the chakras. A tea made with holy basil is also beneficial in aiding meditation and deep personal introspection. As a variety of basil, it is easy to grow and is the perfect addition to any herb garden.

CALMING MASSAGE OIL

When muscles are tight due to tension and stress, reach for this calming massage oil. Sometimes a good neck, shoulder and back massage is what is needed to release unnecessary tension. Have a friend or partner use this sweet-smelling oil to make the experience even more relaxing. Chamomile, lavender and lemon balm are all calming herbs that will also help to soothe sore muscles.

Yield: about ¾ cup (180 ml)

Ingredients
¼ cup (6 g) dried chamomile flowers
2 tbsp (5 g) dried lavender flowers
2 tbsp (4 g) dried lemon balm
½ cup (120 ml) sweet almond oil
¼ cup (60 ml) coconut oil, melted
5–10 drops lavender essential oil (optional)

Instructions
Combine the chamomile, lavender and lemon balm with the sweet almond and coconut oils in a half-pint (236-ml) jar. Cover the jar with a lid and shake to mix well. Put the jar in a cool, dark place to infuse for 4 to 6 weeks. Strain out the plant material with a fine-mesh sieve. If the coconut oil has solidified in the oil infusion, gently heat it by setting the jar in a pan of warm water to melt the oil before straining. Then add the lavender essential oil (if using) and stir well.

Use the oil as often as needed for massage and to aid in relieving muscle tension. If you prefer, the oil can be heated prior to use by placing the jar in a pan of warm water.

This massage oil is safe to use on children ages 1 year and older following a patch test (see page 23). Omit the lavender essential oil for those under age 13.

Tip: Other calming and muscle-soothing herbs that can be used in this massage oil are peppermint, Saint John's wort, ginger, rose petals, geranium flowers, calendula flowers, sage and whole vanilla beans.

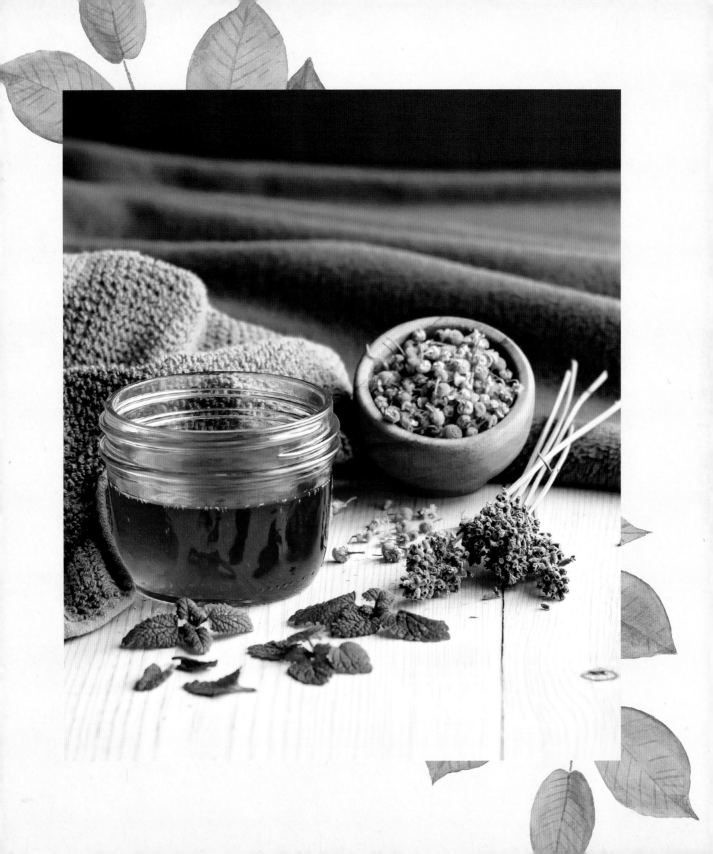

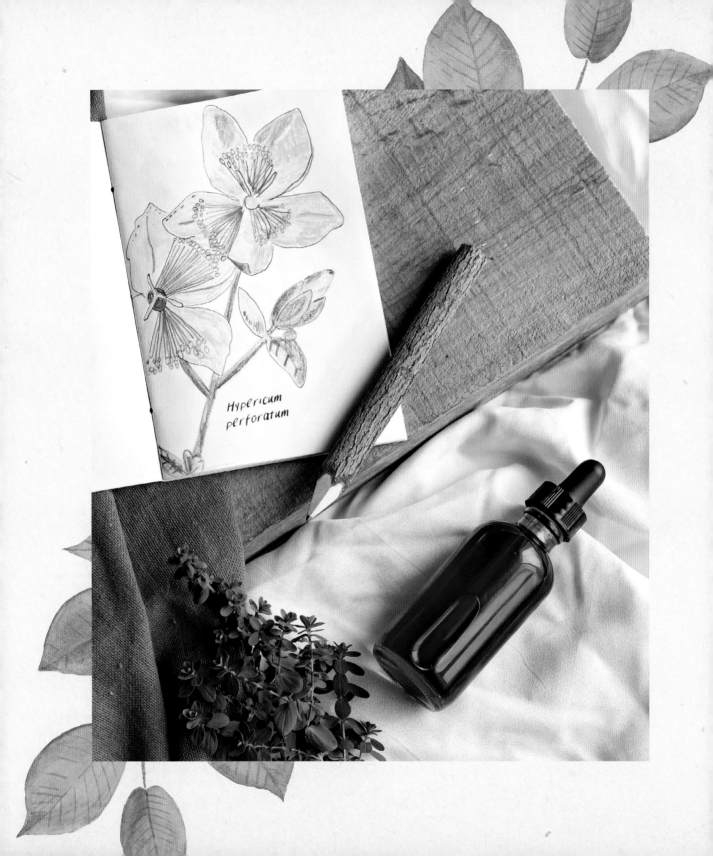

Hypericum
perforatum

SAINT JOHN'S WORT TINCTURE FOR LIFTING LOW SPIRITS

When your spirits are low and feelings of melancholy abound, this Saint John's wort tincture can help. Saint John's wort has been proven to be very effective for treating mild depression, seasonal affective disorder and for when you're generally feeling down. If you have access to fresh Saint John's wort flowers, which are abundant in many areas during the summertime, definitely use them to make this tincture as they lose some of their potency when dried. To experience the most benefit, this tincture is best taken in a cycle of 2 to 3 weeks on, then 1 week off. It may take several weeks to notice an improvement in spirits when taking this tincture. For severe depression, please consult your doctor.

Yield: about ¾ cup (180 ml)

Ingredients
¼ cup (15 g) dried or ½ cup (30 g) fresh Saint John's wort flowers and leaves
¾ cup (180 ml) vodka or other neutral spirits

Instructions
Combine the Saint John's wort and spirits in a half-pint (236-ml) jar, then cover with a lid. Put the jar in a cool, dark place to infuse for 4 to 6 weeks. When ready to use, strain out the herbs with a fine-mesh sieve. Store the tincture in small bottles with droppers for easy use.

Take 1 teaspoon (5 ml) twice daily as a mood enhancer and to mitigate the effects of depression for 2 to 3 weeks, then take 1 week off before repeating the cycle again.

For children and those wishing to avoid alcohol, this tincture can be made with vegetable glycerine instead of the neutral spirits. If made in this manner, it is safe for children ages 8 and older. Please follow the dosage guidelines on page 23.

Tip: Saint John's wort is often considered a "weed" because it grows without abandon in the summertime. As with many weeds, this one is highly useful to us for so many things, so it is a good one to learn how to identify when you're out wildcrafting. Collect the little yellow flowers when you see them for use in this tincture and for the Saint John's Wort & Cayenne Warming Oil recipe on page 53.

CALIFORNIA POPPY TINCTURE FOR RELAXATION

Poppies are a lovely flower that have profound relaxation properties. Remember Dorothy from the *Wizard of Oz* falling asleep in a field of poppies? There was a bit of truth to that scene. Opium, a powerful pain-relieving narcotic, is derived from the opium poppy. California poppy, a beautiful bright orange flower that grows in the southwestern United States and parts of Mexico, isn't nearly as strong as opium, but still has some wonderful and relaxing effects in a whole plant form that is much more gentle. It also reduces stress and helps to bring on sleep.

Yield: about ¾ cup (180 ml)

Ingredients
½ cup (8 g) loosely packed, dried California poppy flowers, leaves and stems
¾ cup (180 ml) vodka or other neutral spirits

Instructions
Combine the California poppy and spirits in a half-pint (236-ml) jar, then cover with a lid. Put the jar in a cool, dark place to infuse for 4 to 6 weeks. When ready to use, strain out the herbs with a fine-mesh sieve. Store the tincture in small bottles with droppers for easy use.

Take ½ to 1 teaspoon (2 to 5 ml) daily to relax, ease stress or as a natural sleep aid.

For children and those wishing to avoid alcohol, this tincture can be made with vegetable glycerine instead of the neutral spirits. If made in this manner, it is safe for children ages 8 and older. Please follow the dosing guidelines on page 23.

Tip: There is a big misconception that it is illegal to pick California poppies in the state of California, where it is the state flower. In fact, it's only illegal to pick them on state or federal land, which is the case for any plant or flower, not only for poppies. This means that if you are in California and not on federal or state land, it is perfectly fine to forage for California poppies, which set the hillsides ablaze with bright orange in springtime.

Healing Herbal Infusions

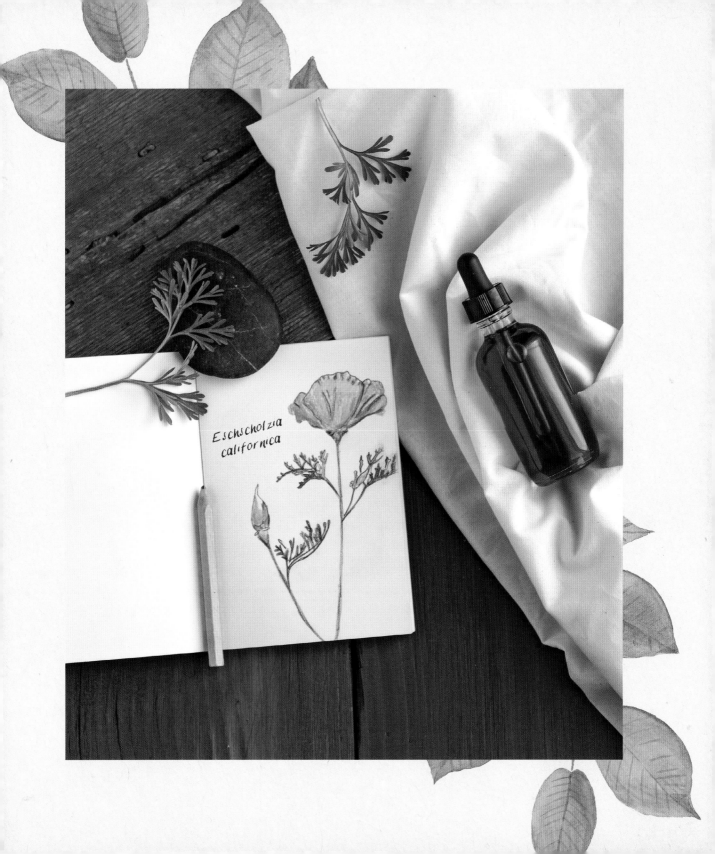

Eschscholzia
californica

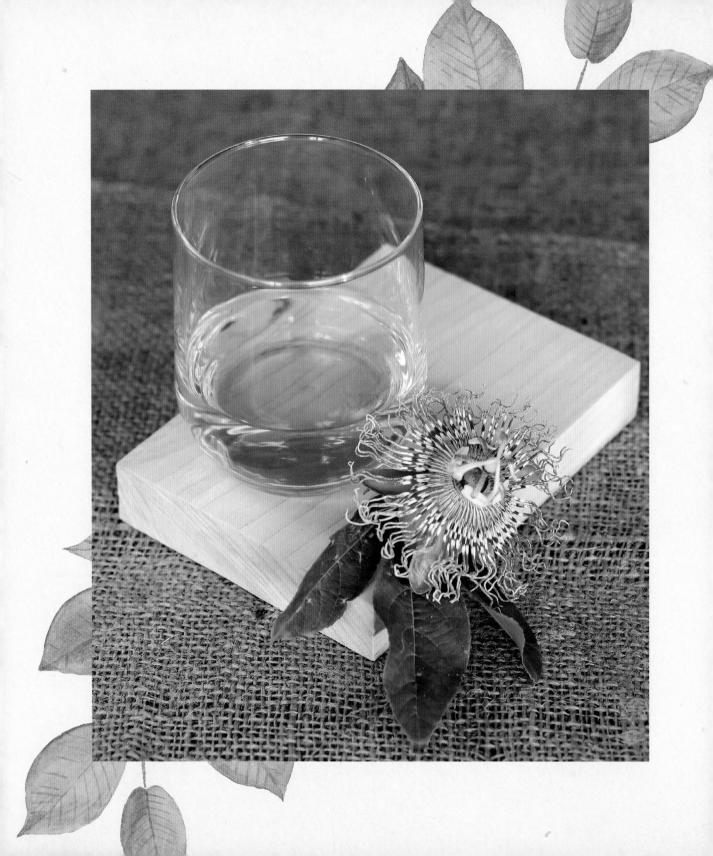

PASSIONFLOWER-INFUSED WINE

Passiflora, also known as passionflower, is a tropical vining plant with truly wonderful and unique flowers. They are gorgeous, delicate-looking flowers without being fragile at all. Passionflower vines are easy to grow in your garden and can also be foraged in the southeastern United States and parts of Mexico and South America where they grow wild. They are calming and relaxing to the nervous system, helping to reduce anxiety and overstimulation. Infusing fresh passionflowers into wine is a nice way to enjoy their benefits. This infused wine is to be thought of as medicine, and no more than one small glass should be consumed per day.

Yield: about 1¾ cups (420 ml)

Ingredients
½ oz (14 g) fresh passionflowers
1¾ cups (420 ml) white wine

Instructions
Combine the passionflowers and wine in a pint-size (473-ml) jar, then cover with a lid. Put the jar in a cool, dark place to infuse for 4 to 6 weeks. When ready to use, strain out the flowers with a fine-mesh sieve.

Drink one 4-ounce (120-ml) glass to help relax and to bring on sleep.

Infused wine is not meant to be consumed by anyone under the legal drinking age.

Tip: Take all of your wine to the next level by infusing it with flowers! Here are some other flowers that are wonderful when infused into wine: lavender, chamomile, elderflower, hibiscus, rose petals, violets, honeysuckle and red clover.

REJUVENATING FLOWER BATH SOAK

A hot mineral bath can do wonders for the soul, not to mention relax the muscles and help to ease tension. Epsom salt is high in magnesium, a vital mineral that many of us are lacking, which is best absorbed through the skin. Magnesium is good for so many things, namely easing sore muscles and promoting restful sleep. A blend of lavender, chamomile and rose petals make for a calming and rejuvenating bath-time experience with their pleasant scent.

Yield: 1¾ cups (276 g)

Ingredients
1 cup (260 g) Epsom salt
¼ cup (9 g) dried lavender flowers
¼ cup (5 g) dried chamomile flowers
¼ cup (2 g) dried rose petals

Instructions
Combine the Epsom salt and the dried flowers in a small bowl and stir to combine, then transfer to a jar with a lid.

When ready to use, fill a large reusable muslin bag or a piece of cheesecloth tied with a string with ¼ to ½ cup (40 to 80 g) of the salt and flower mixture. Add it to a hot bath. The salt will dissolve, and the flowers will stay in the muslin bag and infuse into the bathwater.

This bath soak is safe to use for children ages 2 years and older following a patch test (see page 23).

Tip: Other flowers that would work in this recipe are elderflower, geranium and violets. For a more invigorating bath soak, swap out the flowers for peppermint, rosemary and orange peel.

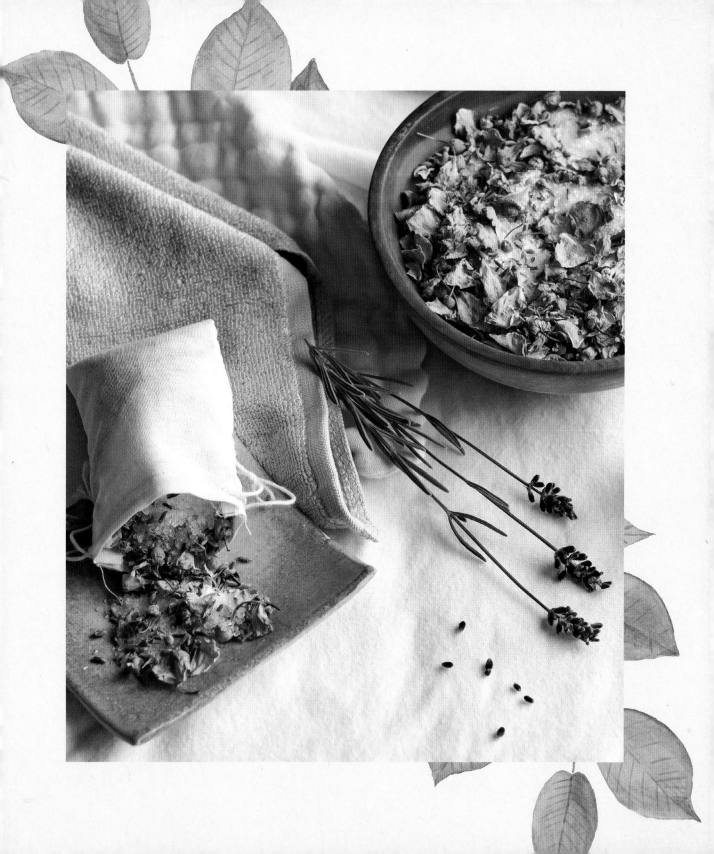

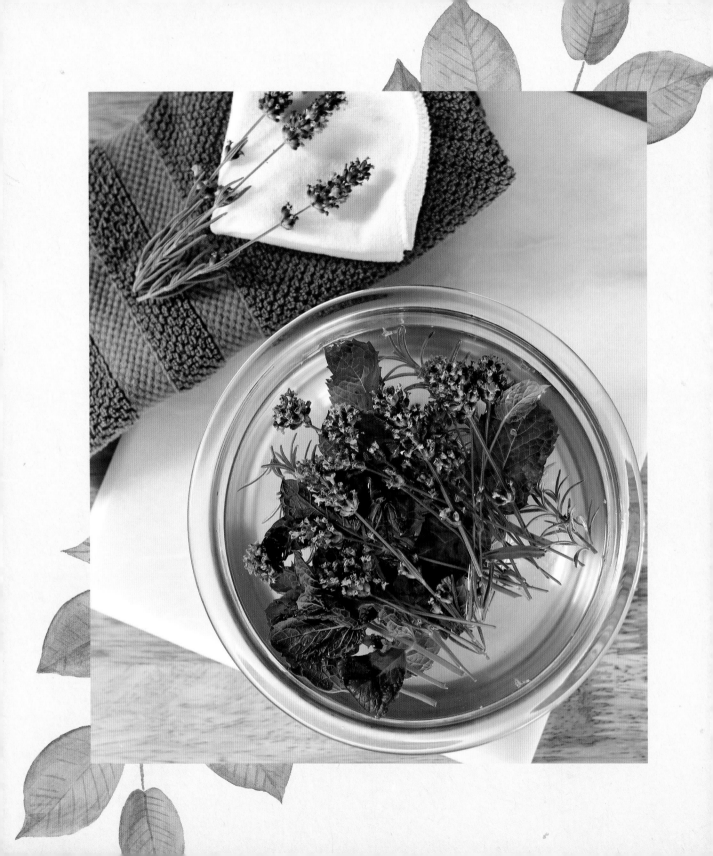

RELAXING HERBAL FACE STEAM

For a quick and easy way to relax, try this herbal face steam. The aromatherapy from the herbs will calm your nerves and ease your mind. The steam combined with the volatile oils in the herbs will also help to cleanse and open up the pores in your face. This combination of rosemary, peppermint and lavender smells absolutely amazing and has a powerful relaxation effect. I prefer to use fresh herbs when making herbal face steams because they have more volatile oils, but dried herbs will still be beneficial if that's all you have access to. The addition of eucalyptus essential oil is nice, especially for helping to clear up nasal congestion.

Yield: 1 face steam

Ingredients
6 cups (1½ L) water
½ cup (8 g) loosely packed fresh rosemary
½ cup (8 g) loosely packed fresh peppermint
½ cup (8 g) loosely packed fresh lavender flowers
3–5 drops eucalyptus essential oil (optional)

Instructions
Bring the water to a boil and pour it over the herbs in a medium-size heatproof bowl. Then add the eucalyptus essential oil (if using).

Hang a towel over the back of your head, then lean over the bowl to allow the steam on your face; slowly inhale. If it feels too hot at any moment, remove your face from the bowl.

Repeat once daily for as long as you like to help relax and rejuvenate.

This face steam is safe to use on children ages 8 years and older. Just be extra careful that it isn't too hot.

Tip: Some other great herbs and flowers to use in this face steam are thyme, sage, basil, lemon balm, calendula, rose petals, chamomile and elderflower. If you have access to fresh eucalyptus leaves, you can use them instead of the essential oil.

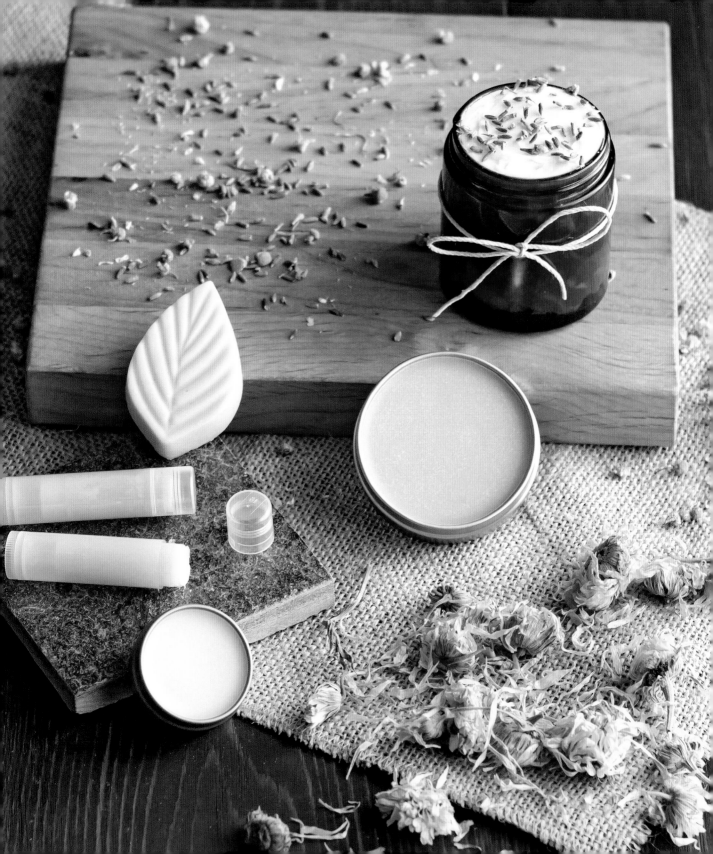

INFUSIONS TO NOURISH YOUR SKIN, LIPS & HAIR

If you've ever wanted to start making your own beauty and skin health-care products with all-natural ingredients to replace chemical-laden conventional products, this is the chapter for you! Many herbs and flowers have amazing skin- and hair-nourishing properties. Calendula flowers are amazing for the skin, and I always (always!) make sure to have calendula infused oil made up at my house for use in recipes. Rose hips, lavender, elderflower, marshmallow root, violet leaf and chickweed are all great for healing and repairing damaged skin, making them stellar ingredients for infused oils, salves, balms, body butters and lotion bars. Rosemary, sage, nettles and mint are beneficial and restorative for the hair, scalp and beard. Help to nourish and repair your skin, lips and hair using all-natural herbal ingredients with these simple recipes.

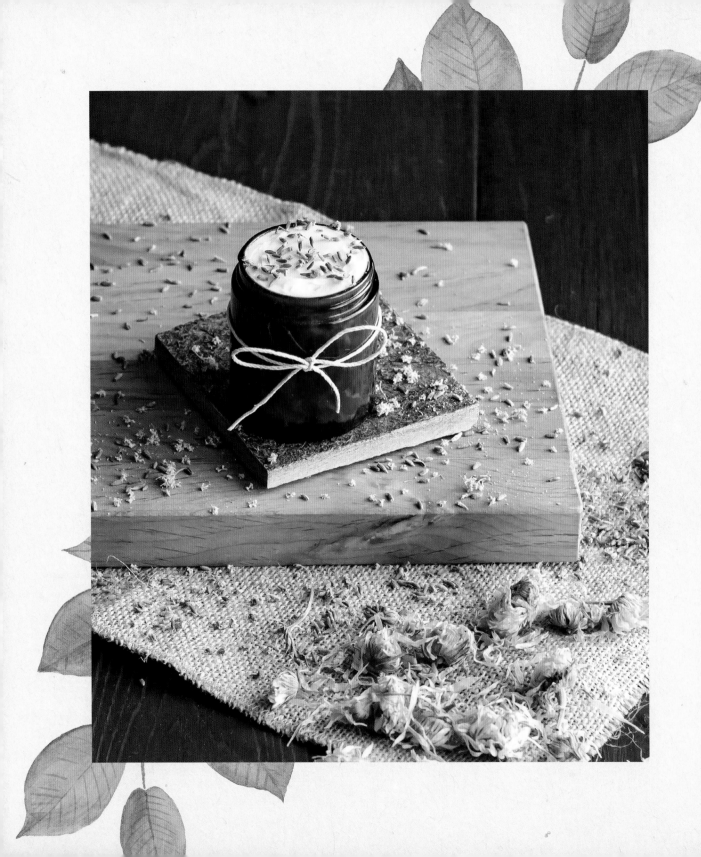

HEALING FLOWER-WHIPPED BODY BUTTER

When you really need a good moisturizer, sometimes a salve just isn't enough. That's where this body butter comes in. It has a good portion of shea butter and coconut oil, plus extra hydrating sweet almond, apricot kernel and castor oils. Calendula flowers are arguably the best herb for skin care and for speeding the healing of bruises, burns, minor wounds and scars. Lavender is anti-inflammatory and has a pleasing scent, and elderflowers promote softer skin. This body butter is sure to be a new favorite!

Yield: about 12 ounces (360 ml) of body butter

Ingredients

For the Infused Oil
¼ cup (5 g) dried calendula flowers
2 tbsp (5 g) dried lavender flowers
2 tbsp (3 g) dried elderflowers
¼ cup (60 ml) coconut oil, melted
¼ cup (60 ml) sweet almond oil

¼ cup (60 ml) apricot kernel oil
1 tbsp (15 ml) castor oil

For the Body Butter
4 oz (112 g) shea butter
½ cup (120 ml) flower-infused oil
5–10 drops lavender essential oil (optional)

Instructions

Combine the calendula, lavender and elderflowers with the coconut, sweet almond, apricot kernel and castor oils in a half-pint (236-ml) jar. Cover the jar with a lid and shake to mix well. Put the jar in a cool, dark place to infuse for 4 to 6 weeks.

When you are ready to make the body butter, strain the flowers from the oil using a fine-mesh sieve. If the coconut oil has solidified in the oil infusion, gently heat it by setting the jar in a pan of warm water to melt the oil before straining. Measure out ½ cup (120 ml) of the infused oil and set aside.

Put the shea butter into a double boiler on medium heat (see tips for making your own double boiler on page 20) until it has completely melted, then promptly remove from the heat. Add the flower-infused oil and the lavender essential oil (if using) to the melted shea butter and stir to combine. Pour the mixture into a medium-size mixing bowl and put in the refrigerator until it just begins to solidify, about 1 hour.

Remove the mixture from the refrigerator, and use a hand blender to whip the mixture for several minutes into a light and smooth butter. Scrape the body butter out of the bowl and into jars or tins for storage.

Apply the body butter as often as needed to help moisturize the skin and to heal minor skin issues.

This body butter is safe to use on children ages 1 year and older following a patch test (see page 23). Omit the lavender essential oil for those under age 13.

ROSE PETAL & ROSE HIP FACE SERUM

With aging skin comes unwanted wrinkles, sun spots and scars. Many store-bought skin care products for the face have less than ideal ingredients, but thankfully it is easy to make your own. Rose hip seed oil is high in antioxidants and essential fatty acids, and it is known for its anti-aging effects, helping to smooth wrinkles and fade sun spots and scars. Even young and healthy skin can benefit from rose hip seed oil, as it is a highly effective facial moisturizer that doesn't leave behind any greasiness. When combined and infused with rose petals and rose hips, it makes a triple rose serum that is perfect for using on the face.

Yield: about ½ cup (120 ml)

Ingredients
½ cup (120 ml) rose hip seed oil

¼ cup (2 g) dried rose petals

2 tbsp (15 g) dried rose hips

Instructions
Combine the rose hip seed oil, rose petals and rose hips in a half-pint (236-ml) jar. Cover the jar with a lid and shake to mix well. Put the jar in a cool, dark place to infuse for 4 to 6 weeks. When ready to use, strain out the herbs with a fine-mesh sieve.

Apply a small amount of the oil on the face and neck daily to hydrate, improve skin tone and fade wrinkles.

This face serum is safe to use on children ages 2 years and older following a patch test (see page 23).

Tip: Rose hip seed oil is sensitive to light and heat, so it is helpful to store it in an amber bottle in a cool location. In the summer months, you may want to store this infusion in the refrigerator.

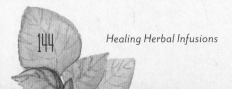

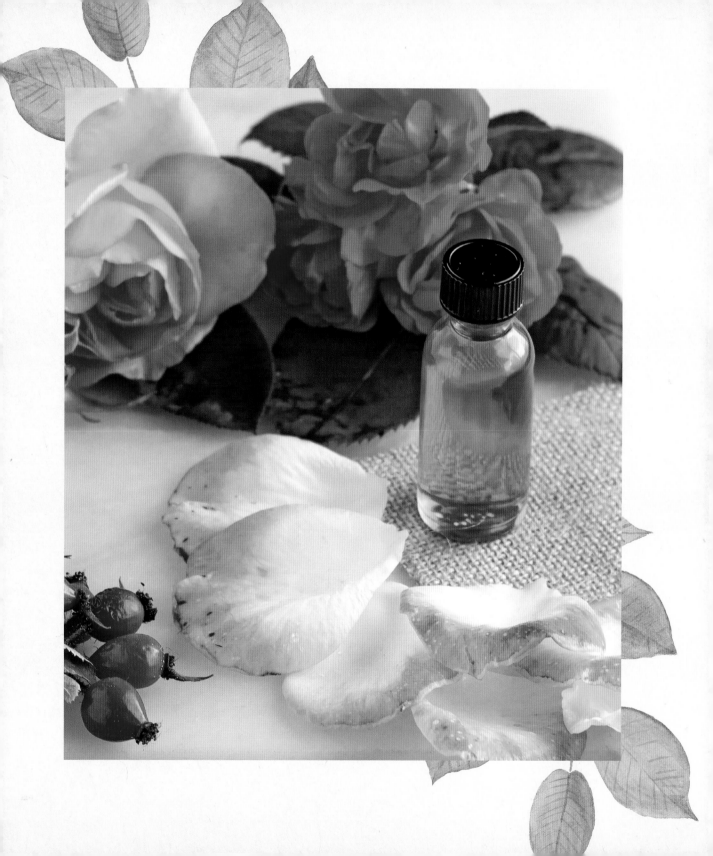

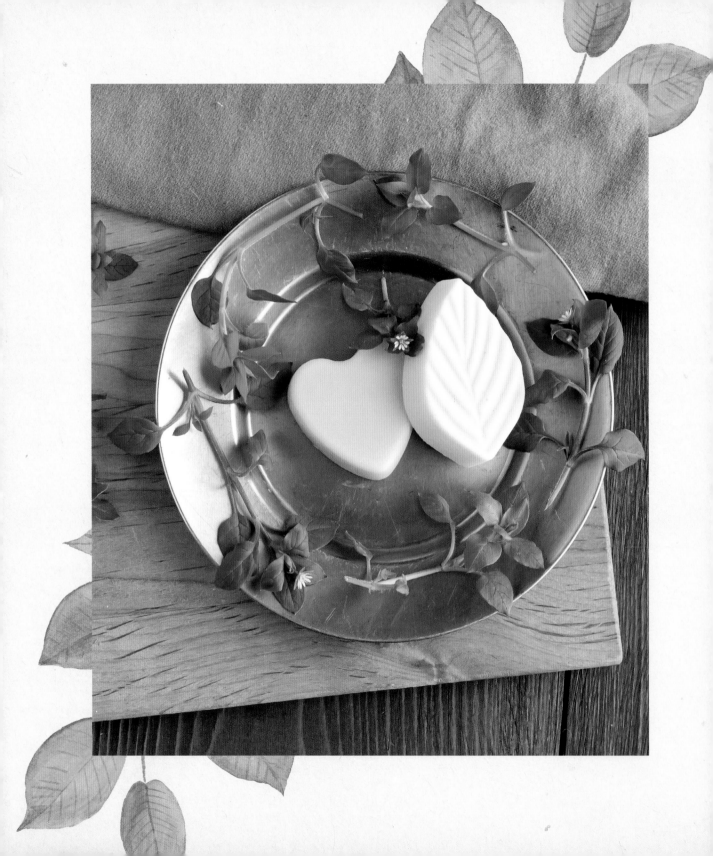

SOOTHING CHICKWEED LOTION BARS

For very dry, calloused and cracked skin, lotion bars can't be beat. They coat the affected area well and the moisturizing effect lasts for hours, plus their portability makes them very easy to always have on hand. Chickweed is a particularly soothing herb for extra dry skin due to its mucilaginous properties. It is a common "weed" that makes an appearance in the early spring in many locations and is easy to forage for. These lotion bars are popular with men because they repair and soften calluses and cracked fingertips quickly and don't have a "flowery" scent.

Yield: about 5–6 lotion bars, if using a mold with 2-ounce (60-ml) cups

Ingredients

For the Infused Oil
½ cup (15 g) dried chickweed
¼ cup (60 ml) coconut oil, melted
¼ cup (60 ml) olive oil
¼ cup (60 ml) sweet almond oil

For the Lotion Bars
½ cup chickweed-infused oil
3 oz (85 g) beeswax
4 oz (113 g) shea butter

Instructions

Combine the chickweed with the coconut, olive and sweet almond oils in a half-pint (236-ml) jar. Cover the jar with a lid and shake to mix well. Put the jar in a cool, dark place to infuse for 4 to 6 weeks.

When you are ready to make the lotion bars, strain the herb from the oil using a fine-mesh sieve. If the coconut oil has solidified in the oil infusion, gently heat it by setting the jar in a pan of warm water to melt the oil before straining. Measure out ½ cup (120 ml) of the infused oil, saving any excess oil for later use if you wish. Put the oil into a double boiler on medium heat (see tips for making your own double boiler on page 20). Add the beeswax to the oil and continue to heat until it has completely melted. Next, add the shea butter, and when it has melted, remove the mixture from the heat. Carefully pour the mixture into a lotion bar or soap mold. Let the lotion bars cool and set up for 3 to 4 hours before removing them from the mold.

To use, rub the lotion bar on areas of dry skin as often as needed.

These lotion bars are safe to use on children ages 1 year and older following a patch test (see page 23).

Tip: Lotion bars can be made with many different skin-healing herbs and flowers. Some of my favorites are calendula, violet leaf, rose petals, lavender and dandelion.

DRY HANDS BALM

This soothing balm is made especially for repairing and moisturizing very dry hands. Violet leaf and chickweed are excellent hydrating herbs, and lavender is healing and has a pleasant smell. Sweet almond and apricot kernel oils are emollient without being greasy, and castor oil and mango butter are both rich and skin softening. Reach for this balm when the weather is dry and your hands and fingertips could use a little extra love.

Yield: about 6 ounces (180 ml) of balm

Ingredients

For the Infused Oil
2 tbsp (4 g) dried chickweed
2 tbsp (8 g) dried violet leaf
¼ cup (8 g) dried lavender flowers
¼ cup (60 ml) olive oil
¼ cup (60 ml) sweet almond oil
¼ cup (60 ml) apricot kernel oil
1 tbsp (15 ml) castor oil

For the Balm
½ cup (120 ml) infused oil
½ oz (14 g) beeswax
1 oz (28 g) mango butter
8 drops lavender essential oil

Instructions

Combine the chickweed, violet leaf and lavender with the olive, sweet almond, apricot kernel and castor oils in a half-pint (236-ml) jar. Cover the jar with a lid and shake to mix well. Put the jar in a cool, dark place to infuse for 4 to 6 weeks.

When you are ready to make the balm, strain the herbs from the oil using a fine-mesh sieve. Measure out ½ cup (120 ml) of the infused oil, saving any excess oil for later use if you wish. Put the oil into a double boiler on medium heat (see tips for making your own double boiler on page 20). Add the beeswax to the oil and continue to heat until it has completely melted. Next, add the mango butter, and when it has melted, remove the mixture from the heat. Carefully pour the mixture into jars or tins. Let the balm cool and set up for 3 to 4 hours before use.

Apply as often as needed to soften and moisturize dry hands.

This hand balm is safe to use on children ages 1 year and older following a patch test (see page 23). Omit the lavender essential oil for those under age 13.

Healing Herbal Infusions

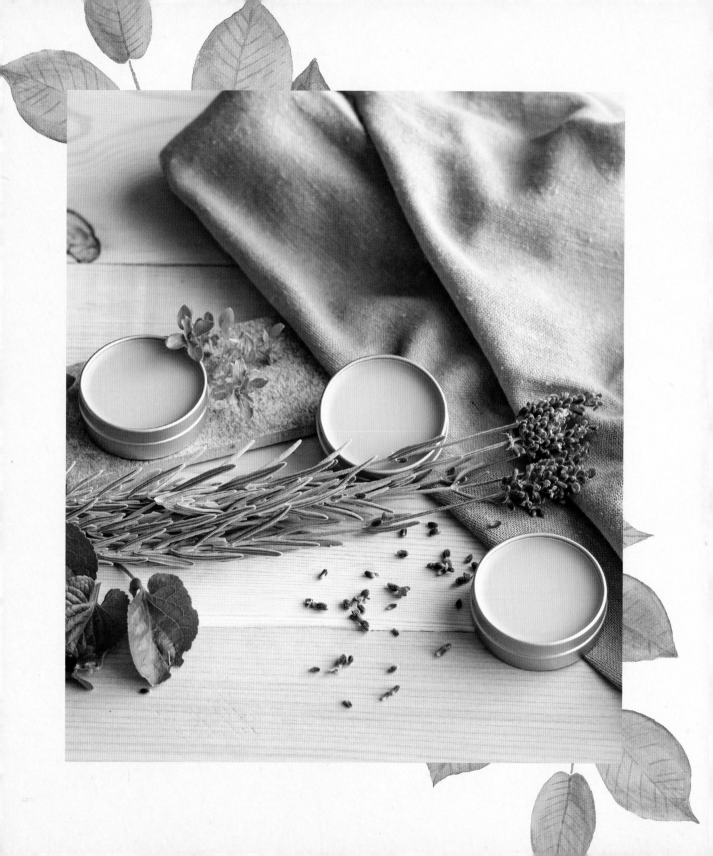

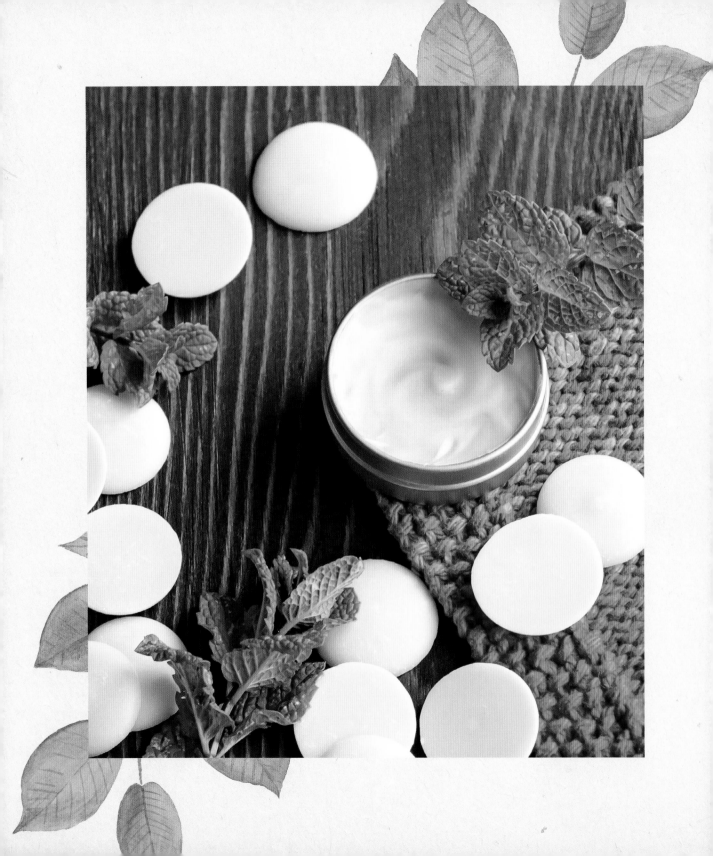

COCOA MINT CRACKED HEEL BALM

When the weather is cold and dry, cracked heels can be a painful problem that is hard to fix. Cocoa butter comes to the rescue here, as it is super moisturizing and can help to repair very dry and cracked feet. Marshmallow root is mucilaginous, making it soothing and healing for cracked skin. Using unrefined cocoa butter in this recipe gives it that characteristic chocolate aroma, which pairs nicely with the peppermint. If you want all the benefits of cocoa butter without the scent, use a naturally refined version.

Yield: about 6 ounces (180 ml) of balm

Ingredients

For the Infused Oil
¼ cup (5 g) dried calendula flowers
2 tbsp (5 g) dried marshmallow root
2 tbsp (5 g) dried peppermint
¼ cup (60 ml) coconut oil, melted
¼ cup (60 ml) olive oil
¼ cup (60 ml) sweet almond oil
1 tbsp (15 ml) castor oil

For the Balm
½ cup (120 ml) infused oil
½ oz (14 g) beeswax
1 oz (28 g) unrefined cocoa butter
8 drops peppermint essential oil

Instructions

Combine the calendula, marshmallow root and peppermint with the coconut, olive, sweet almond and castor oils in a half-pint (236-ml) jar. Cover the jar with a lid and shake to mix well. Put the jar in a cool, dark place to infuse for 4 to 6 weeks.

When you are ready to make the balm, strain the herbs from the oil using a fine-mesh sieve. If the coconut oil has solidified in the oil infusion, gently heat it by setting the jar in a pan of warm water to melt the oil before straining. Measure out ½ cup (120 ml) of the infused oil, saving any excess oil for later use if you wish. Put the oil into a double boiler on medium heat (see tips for making your own double boiler on page 20). Add the beeswax to the oil and continue to heat until it has completely melted. Next, add the cocoa butter, and when it has melted, remove the mixture from the heat. Stir in the peppermint essential oil. Carefully pour the mixture into jars or tins. Let the balm cool and set up for 3 to 4 hours before use.

Apply as often as needed to soften dry feet and repair cracked heels.

This foot balm is safe to use on children ages 1 year and older following a patch test (see page 23). Omit the peppermint essential oil for those under age 13.

CHAMOMILE, MARSHMALLOW & VANILLA CHAPPED LIP BALM

Chapped lips are a common problem during the winter, especially if you are out in the elements participating in winter activities. This is my absolute favorite lip balm for healing and repairing dry, chapped and cracked lips. Chamomile flowers are calming to the skin with anti-inflammatory properties, and marshmallow root is a powerful natural moisturizer that is very soothing on chapped lips. The addition of a whole vanilla bean provides a wonderful scent that pairs nicely with the chamomile.

Yield: about 6 ounces (180 ml) of lip balm

Ingredients

For the Infused Oil
¼ cup (6 g) dried chamomile flowers

¼ cup (10 g) dried marshmallow root

1 whole vanilla bean, split in half lengthwise

½ cup (120 ml) coconut oil, melted

¼ cup (60 ml) sweet almond oil

1 tbsp (15 ml) castor oil

For the Lip Balm
½ cup (120 ml) infused oil

1 oz (28 g) beeswax

½ oz (14 g) shea butter

Instructions

Combine the chamomile, marshmallow root and vanilla bean with the coconut, sweet almond and castor oils in a half-pint (236-ml) jar. Cover the jar with a lid and shake to mix well. Put the jar in a cool, dark place to infuse for 4 to 6 weeks.

When you are ready to make the lip balm, strain the herbs from the oil using a fine-mesh sieve. If the coconut oil has solidified in the oil infusion, gently heat it by setting the jar in a pan of warm water to melt the oil before straining. Measure out ½ cup (120 ml) of the infused oil, saving any excess oil for later use if you wish. Put the oil into a double boiler on medium heat (see tips for making your own double boiler on page 20). Add the beeswax to the oil and continue to heat until it has completely melted. Next, add the shea butter, and when it has melted, remove the mixture from the heat. Carefully pour the mixture into small tins or lip balm tubes. Let the lip balm cool and set up for 3 to 4 hours before use.

Apply as often as needed to soften and repair chapped lips.

This lip balm is safe to use on children ages 2 years and older following a patch test (see page 23).

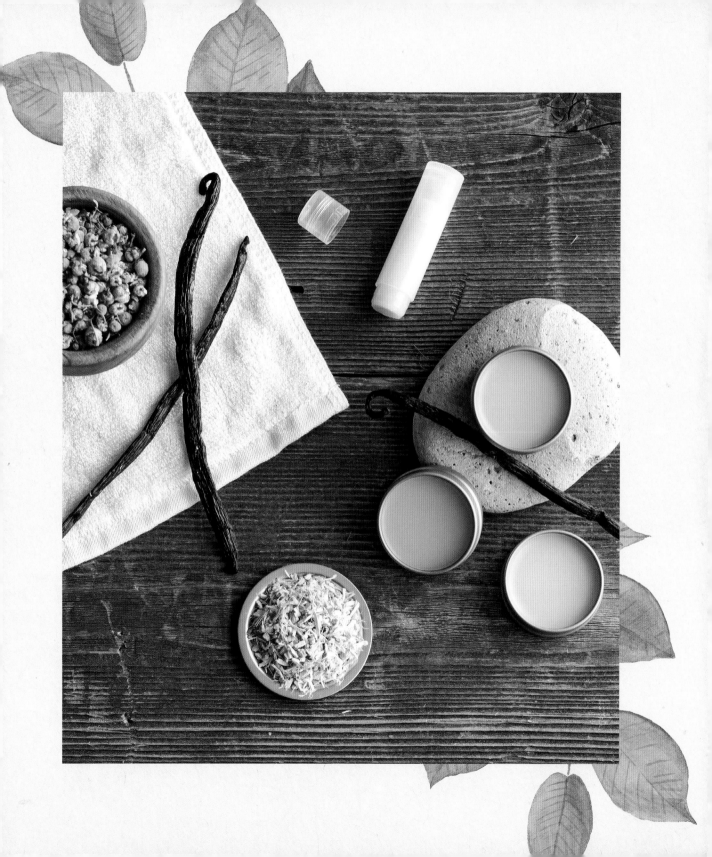

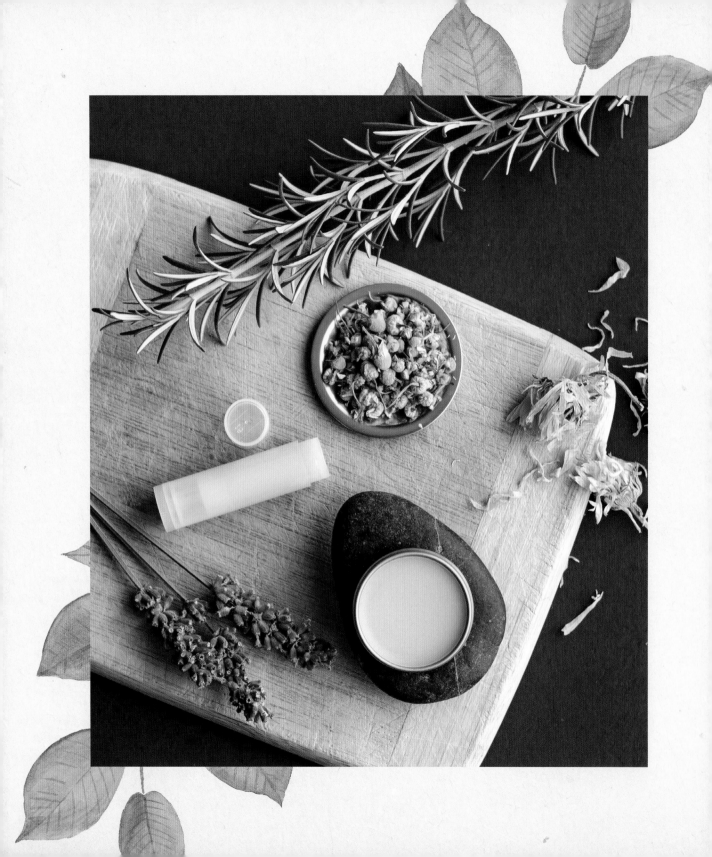

BLEMISH BALM

There is nothing more annoying than an unexpected pimple. This blemish balm contains three intense skin-healing flowers: calendula, lavender and chamomile. They work quickly to reduce the redness and pain associated with pimples and acne. Tea tree and rosemary essential oils are highly beneficial for treating pimples and can almost eliminate them within a day or two. For super easy application and portability, try using lip balm tubes for this blemish balm. This balm is ideal for those with dry to normal complexions. If you have oily skin, substitute the coconut oil with a greater portion of sweet almond or apricot kernel oil; they are much lighter on the skin.

Yield: about 5 ounces (150 ml) of balm

Ingredients

For the Infused Oil
¼ cup (5 g) dried calendula flowers

2 tbsp (5 g) dried lavender flowers

2 tbsp (3 g) dried chamomile flowers

¼ cup (60 ml) coconut oil, melted

¼ cup (60 ml) sweet almond oil

¼ cup (60 ml) apricot kernel oil

For the Balm
½ cup (120 ml) infused oil

½ oz (14 g) beeswax (double the amount if using tubes)

½ oz (14 g) shea butter

10 drops tea tree essential oil

10 drops rosemary essential oil

Instructions

Combine the calendula, lavender and chamomile with the coconut, sweet almond and apricot kernel oils in a half-pint (236-ml) jar. Cover the jar with a lid and shake to mix well. Put the jar in a cool, dark place to infuse for 4 to 6 weeks.

When you are ready to make the balm, strain the herbs from the oil using a fine-mesh sieve. If the coconut oil has solidified in the oil infusion, gently heat it by setting the jar in a pan of warm water to melt the oil before straining. Measure out ½ cup (120 ml) of the infused oil, saving any excess oil for later use if you wish. Put the oil into a double boiler on medium heat (see tips for making your own double boiler on page 20). Add the beeswax to the oil and continue to heat until it has completely melted. Next, add the shea butter, and when it has melted, remove the mixture from the heat. Stir in the tea tree and rosemary essential oils. Carefully pour the mixture into small tins or lip balm tubes for easy application. Let the balm cool and set up for 3 to 4 hours before use.

Apply as often as needed to help speed the healing of pimples and blemishes.

This blemish balm is safe to use on children ages 13 and older following a patch test (see page 23).

WITCH HAZEL & BLACKBERRY LEAF FACE WASH

Many over-the-counter face washes have an astringent component because it helps to cleanse the face of dirt and oil buildup and also closes pores and tightens the skin. The good news is that there are herbs that have astringent properties due to naturally occurring tannins, such as witch hazel and blackberry leaf. These herbs also have the added benefit of being anti-inflammatory and having a plethora of skin-healing antioxidants. This herbal face wash can be used like any regular store-bought face wash to remove dirt and make up, but will not be soapy or foam up. The best part is that it is inexpensive and super easy to make at home!

Yield: about 2 cups (480 ml)

Ingredients
2 cups (480 ml) water
2 tbsp (2 g) dried witch hazel
2 tbsp (2 g) dried blackberry leaf

Instructions
Bring the water to a boil and pour it over the herbs in a pint-size (473-ml) mason jar. Let the infusion steep and completely cool to room temperature, then strain out the herbs before using.

Use daily as needed as an astringent and toning face cleanser. Store it in the refrigerator and it will last for up to 1 week. If desired, you can follow up this face wash with the Rose Petal & Rose Hip Face Serum (page 144) for a moisturizing effect.

This face wash is safe to use on children ages 13 and older following a patch test (see page 23).

Tip: Interestingly enough, beyond use as a face wash, these astringent herbs are also highly effective at relieving hemorrhoids. Witch hazel is the main ingredient in many over-the-counter preparations, but making the infusion yourself is simple and much more potent, providing quick relief.

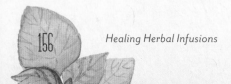

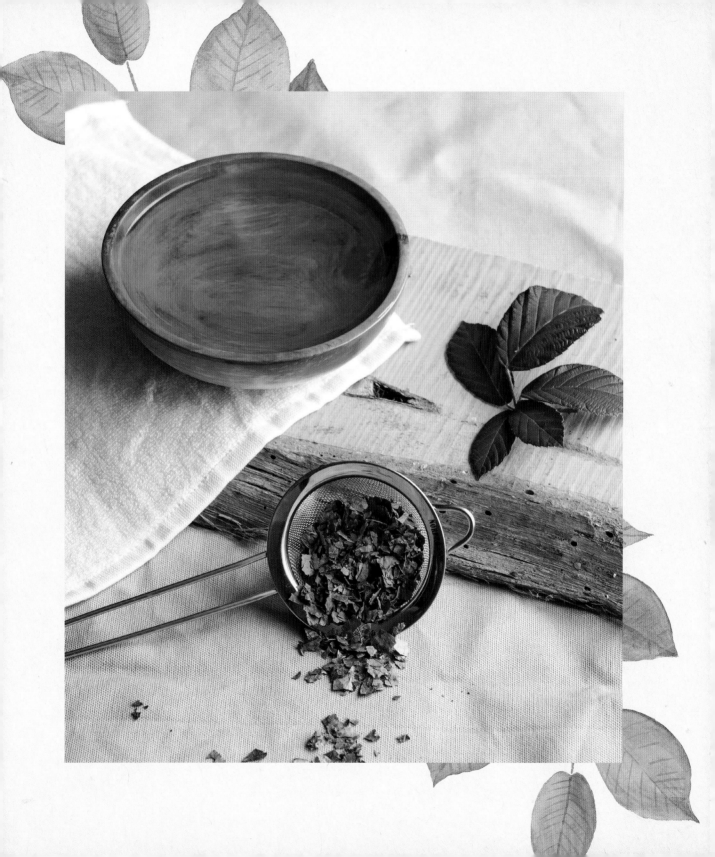

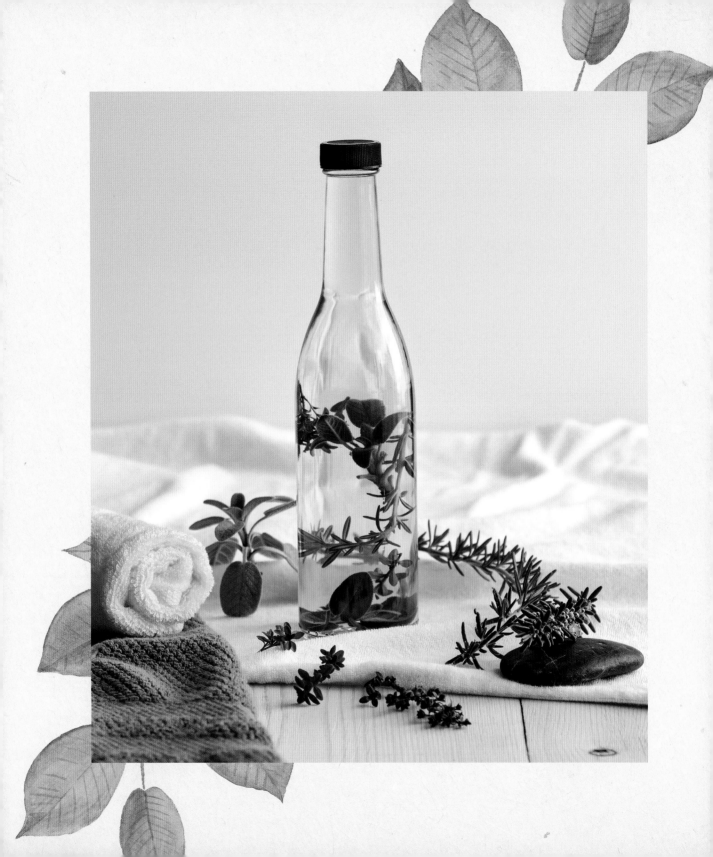

HERBAL HAIR WASH

Using regular shampoo daily can actually be damaging to the hair and scalp. In fact, many naturally minded folks have stopped using shampoo altogether, a practice lovingly called "no poo." This alone can do wonders, but it is still important to nourish and cleanse the hair and scalp occasionally with natural ingredients. Even if you don't want to ditch your shampoo for good, this herbal hair wash is great to use in between regular wash days. Fresh herbs from the garden such as sage, rosemary and thyme have powerful antibacterial and antioxidant properties that are beneficial for the hair. A little bit of baking soda can be added for a deeper cleanse and pairs well when using a vinegar rinse.

Yield: about 2 cups (480 ml)

Ingredients
2 cups (480 ml) water
¼ cup (4 g) loosely packed fresh sage
¼ cup (4 g) loosely packed fresh rosemary
¼ cup (2 g) loosely packed fresh thyme
2 tbsp (30 g) baking soda (optional)

Instructions
Bring the water to a boil and pour it over the herbs in a pint-size (473-ml) mason jar. Let the infusion steep and completely cool to room temperature, then strain out the herbs and stir in the baking soda (if using).

Apply to the hair and massage into the scalp 1 to 2 times per week to cleanse and refresh. This can be followed with a vinegar hair rinse (page 160) if desired.

This hair wash is safe to use on children ages 2 and older following a patch test (see page 23).

Tip: If you'd like to make this hair wash more like a traditional shampoo, add ½ to 1 cup (120 to 240 ml) of liquid castile soap to the infused herbal tea.

SUNFLOWER, VIOLET LEAF & MINT VINEGAR HAIR RINSE

Vinegar rinses are highly beneficial to the hair and scalp by restoring necessary pH. Raw apple cider vinegar is especially nourishing, as it helps to soften the hair and treats a flaky and itchy scalp. When infused with herbs that are known for their hair care properties, you get a powerful rinse that will do wonders for your hair! This vinegar hair rinse can be used after traditional or natural shampoo, shampoo bars or my herbal hair wash recipe on page 159.

Yield: about 2 cups (480 ml)

Ingredients
½ cup (5 g) loosely packed fresh mint leaves
½ cup (7 g) loosely packed fresh violet leaves
½ cup (3 g) fresh or dried sunflower petals
1¾ cups (420 ml) apple cider vinegar
1 cup (240 ml) water (optional)

Instructions
Combine the herbs and apple cider vinegar in a pint-size (473-ml) jar. Cover the jar with a lid, and put in a cool, dark place to infuse for 2 to 6 weeks. Strain out the herbs when ready to use and add the water if you prefer a more diluted vinegar rinse.

Apply to the hair and massage into the scalp 1 to 2 times per week to rinse and refresh the hair and scalp. This can be used after my Herbal Hair Wash (see recipe on page 159).

This hair rinse is safe to use on children ages 2 and older following a patch test (see page 23). I recommend diluting it with water for those under age 13.

Tip: There are many herbs that are beneficial to the hair and scalp that can be substituted if you wish. My favorites are rosemary, sage, thyme, basil, catnip, calendula, chamomile, lavender and nettles.

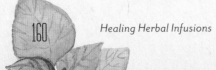

Healing Herbal Infusions

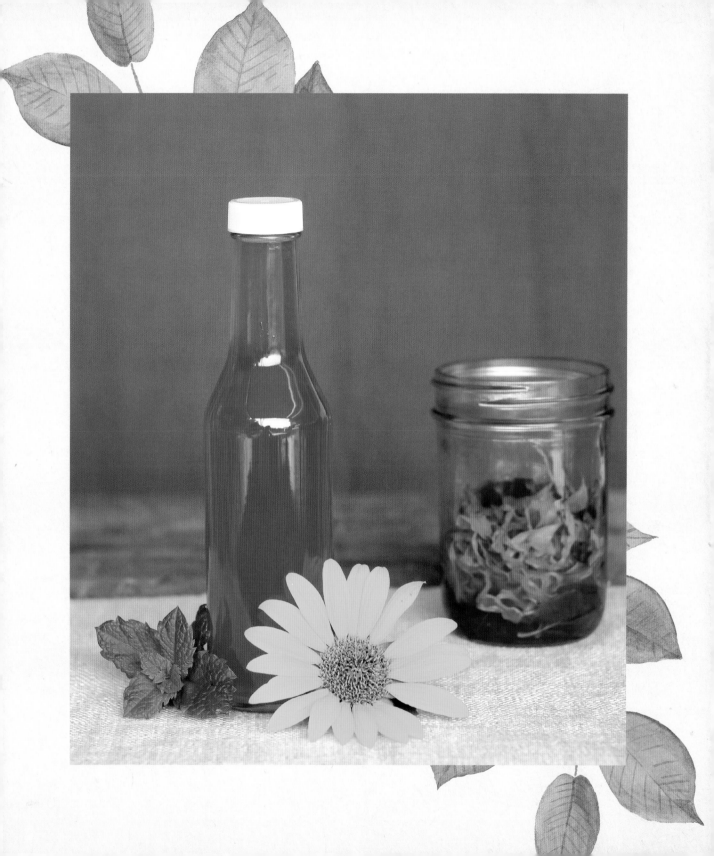

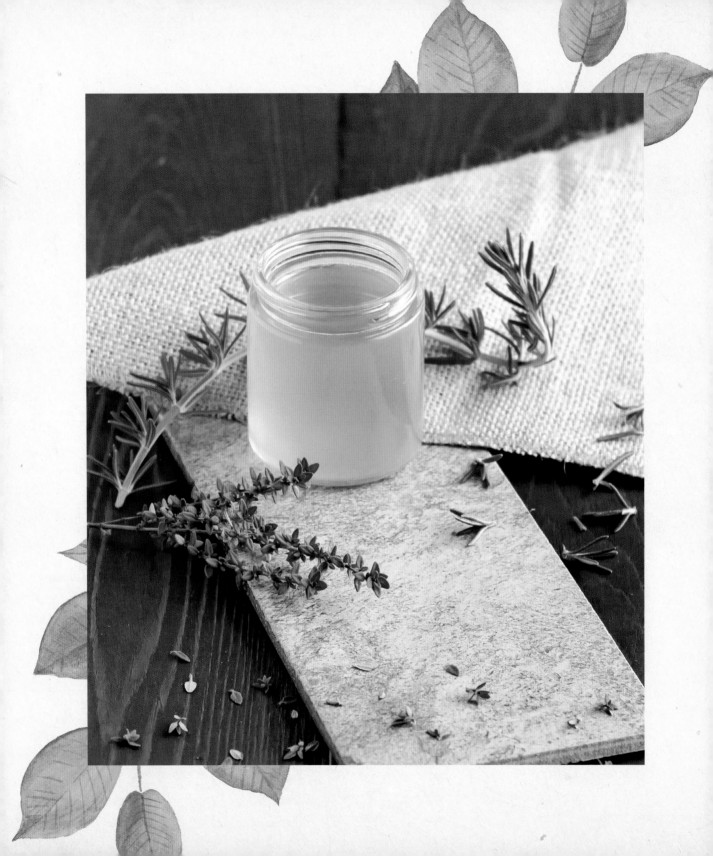

ROSEMARY & THYME FLAKY SCALP TREATMENT

A dry, itchy and flaky scalp is uncomfortable and can be embarrassing. Thankfully, fresh herbs from the garden can come to the rescue! Rosemary and thyme have antibacterial and antifungal properties, and they are excellent for treating a flaky scalp. Coconut oil is moisturizing and hydrating for an irritated scalp, and tea tree essential oil is a powerful antifungal with antiseptic properties. Other herbs that can be used in this remedy are comfrey, sage, catnip, nettles or oregano.

Yield: about ½ cup (120 ml)

Ingredients
2 sprigs (5 g) fresh rosemary
Small bunch (3 g) fresh thyme
½ cup (120 ml) coconut oil
10 drops tea tree essential oil

Instructions
Place the rosemary, thyme and coconut oil into a small saucepan and heat on low for 20 to 30 minutes. Be careful that the oil doesn't become too hot to avoid burning the herbs. Strain out the plant material through a fine-mesh sieve and stir in the tea tree essential oil. Store the oil in a jar covered with a lid. It will solidify at room temperature (below 76°F [24°C]), but will melt on contact with the skin. Because of the herbs' low water content, this oil infusion will last up to 6 months or even longer.

Massage a small amount into a flaky, dry and itchy scalp as often as needed for quick relief and to promote healing. If you find your hair becomes more oily than you like after using this treatment, feel free to follow it with the Herbal Hair Wash (page 159) and Sunflower, Violet Leaf & Mint Vinegar Hair Rinse (page 160) for a full hair and scalp treatment. I recommend leaving this treatment on the scalp for at least 2 hours before rinsing it out, but it can be left on for as long as 24 to 48 hours.

This oil treatment is safe to use on children ages 2 and older following a patch test (see page 23). Omit the tea tree essential oil for those under age 13.

For babies under the age of 2 with cradle cap and other itchy scalp conditions, I recommend using Cradle Cap Oil (page 178).

Tip: This flaky scalp treatment can be made using the long infusion method with dried herbs and with an oil that is liquid at room temperature, such as olive, sweet almond or apricot kernel. Combine the herbs with the oil, cover with a lid and let infuse in a cool, dark place for 4 to 6 weeks. Strain out the herbs and stir in the tea tree oil before using.

SPRUCE & NETTLE BEARD OIL

This oil has a wonderful smell, and it will nourish and repair a dry and scraggly beard. Stinging nettles are highly beneficial for the hair and for dry and flaky skin. Don't worry, there is no sting left in the nettles once they are dried. Jojoba oil is well known for hair repair and is an important addition for moisturizing and hair growth. Spruce cuttings and dried orange peel give this oil a pleasing and manly scent. Feel free to use fresh pine or fir cuttings instead of spruce if that is what you readily have access to.

Yield: about ¾ cup (180 ml)

Ingredients
½ cup (6 g) fresh spruce tips or cuttings

¼ cup (8 g) dried nettles

1 tbsp (8 g) dried orange peel

¼ cup (60 ml) coconut oil, melted

¼ cup (60 ml) olive oil

¼ cup (60 ml) sweet almond oil

2 tbsp (30 ml) jojoba oil

10 drops spruce or fir needle essential oil

5 drops sweet orange essential oil

Instructions
Combine the spruce, nettles and orange peel with the coconut, olive, sweet almond and jojoba oils in a half-pint (236-ml) jar. Cover the jar with a lid and shake to mix well. Put the jar in a cool, dark place to infuse for 4 to 6 weeks. Strain out the plant material with a fine-mesh sieve. If the coconut oil has solidified in the oil infusion, gently heat it by setting the jar in a pan of warm water to melt the oil before straining. Then add the essential oils and stir well.

Use the oil as often as needed to soften and condition the beard.

Tip: This beard oil can also be made into a beard balm if you prefer. Simply melt ¾ ounce (21 g) of beeswax into ½ cup (120 ml) of the strained infused oil over a double boiler and then pour into tins or jars.

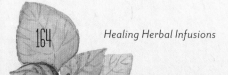

Healing Herbal Infusions

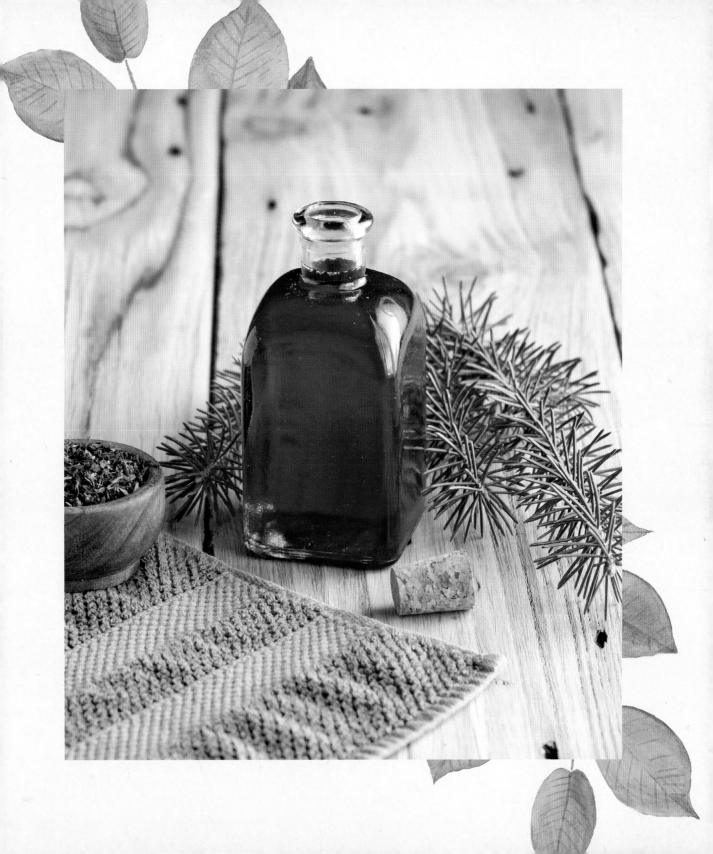

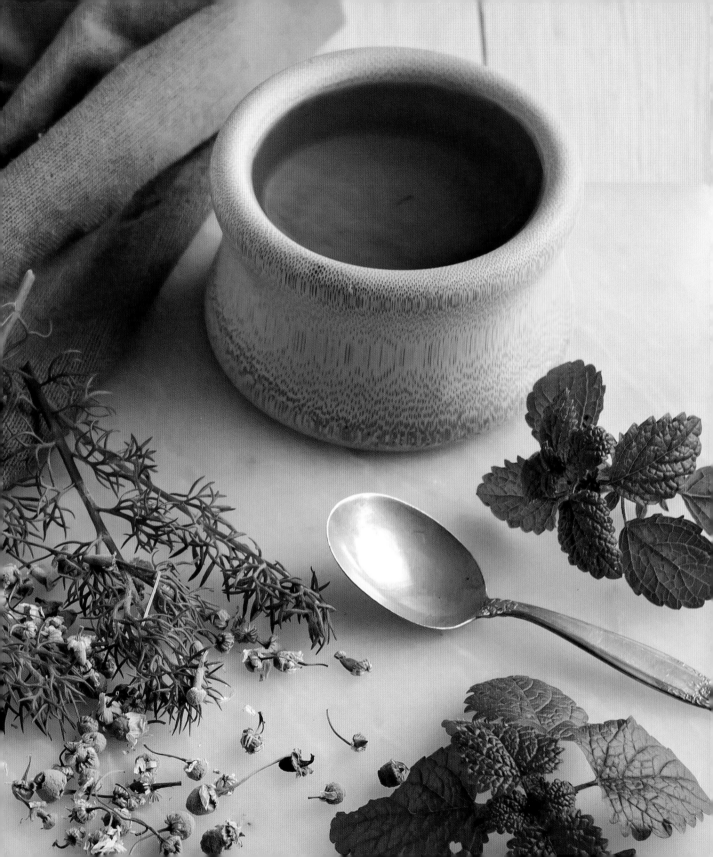

INFUSIONS TO SUPPORT MOTHER & CHILD

Pregnancy is a special time, and great care needs to be taken with what we ingest. Thankfully, there are some safe herbs that can help to support the mother and the growing child. Once that oh-so-beautiful babe arrives, there is a new set of herbs that are gentle enough for the little one, and they are helpful for some common issues that can arise for both mother and infant. There are also a few exceptional herbs to help center, nourish and protect the child as she or he grows, providing calmness and vitality in times of health and sickness. Lemon balm, chamomile, lavender, catnip and calendula are all gentle herbs that are well suited for children and their unique needs.

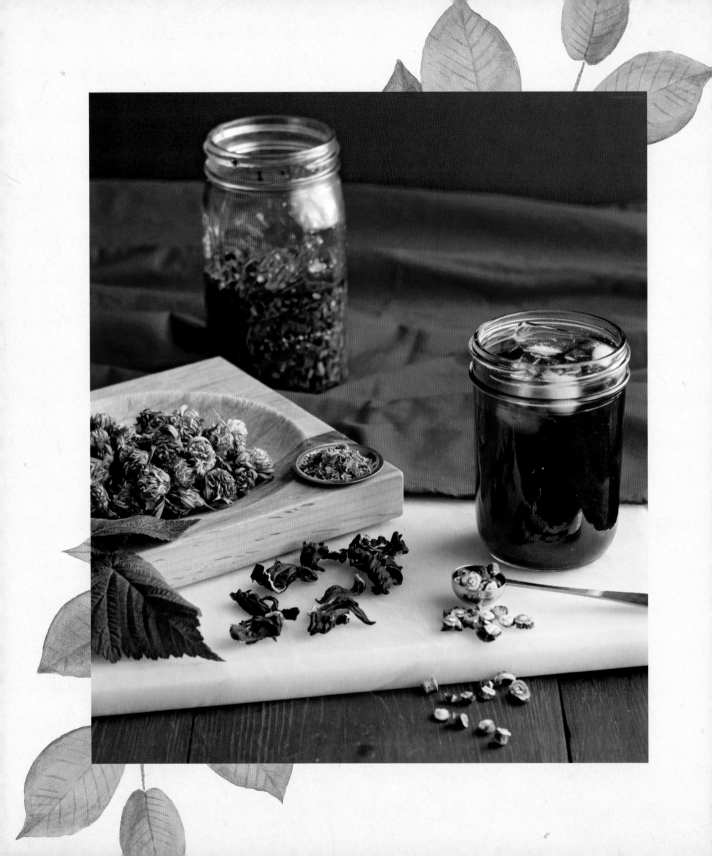

LONG INFUSION FERTILITY TEA

Infertility is unfortunately becoming a common problem in today's world. There are many thoughts on why this may be the case, but whatever the cause, there are herbs that can help. Red clover is a powerful herb to use when preparing for pregnancy, as it is very nourishing to the reproductive system. Red raspberry leaf tones the uterus and gets it ready for supporting a growing baby. Nettles and dandelion root are rich in vitamins and minerals, helping to put the woman in a place of optimum wellness prior to pregnancy. Hibiscus flowers are optional for improving the flavor and adding vitamin C. Please consult with your doctor or midwife before using this infusion, especially if you are on any kind of fertility medication.

Yield: about 4 cups (1 L)

Ingredients
4 cups (1 L) water
½ cup (8 g) dried red clover flowers
½ cup (8 g) dried red raspberry leaf
¼ cup (8 g) dried nettles
1 tbsp (10 g) dried dandelion root
1 tbsp (3 g) dried hibiscus flowers (optional)

Instructions
Bring the water to a boil and pour it over the herbs in a quart-size (946-ml) mason jar. Cover the jar with a lid and let the infusion steep for 4 to 12 hours. Strain with a fine-mesh sieve before drinking. This infusion is best when consumed cold over ice.

Drink 1 to 2 cups (240 to 480 ml) daily in preparation of getting pregnant, ideally for 3 to 6 months prior and while trying to conceive. Discontinue use if you find out you are pregnant.

Tip: This infusion is meant for women, but there are also some beneficial herbs for men's fertility, such as maca root, saw palmetto, tribulus fruit, American ginseng, yohimbe bark and astragalus root.

PREGNANCY TONIC TEA

When I was pregnant, I looked forward to this relaxing cup of tea every evening. It was pleasant on the taste buds and felt very nourishing. Red raspberry leaf is a wonderful herb for supporting pregnancy and toning the uterus, helping to prepare for childbirth and decrease the duration of labor. Peppermint pairs nicely with the red raspberry leaf and can help to ease an upset stomach. Chamomile is relaxing and helps to promote restful sleep. It is best to wait until the second or third trimester to enjoy this tea. Although these herbs are known to be safe to consume while pregnant, it's always best to consult with your doctor or midwife before taking any herbs during pregnancy.

Yield: about 2 cups (480 ml)

Ingredients
2 cups (480 ml) water
2 tbsp (2 g) dried red raspberry leaf
1 tbsp (3 g) dried peppermint
1 tbsp (1 g) dried chamomile flowers

Instructions
Bring the water to a boil and pour over the herbs. Let the infusion steep for 10 to 15 minutes, then strain out the herbs before drinking. This tea can be consumed hot or iced.

Drink 1 to 2 cups (240 to 480 ml) daily during the second and third trimesters to promote a healthy pregnancy, tone the uterus and calm the stomach.

Tip: If you are experiencing acid reflux, which is common during pregnancy, try adding a tablespoon (9 g) of minced fresh ginger to this tea.

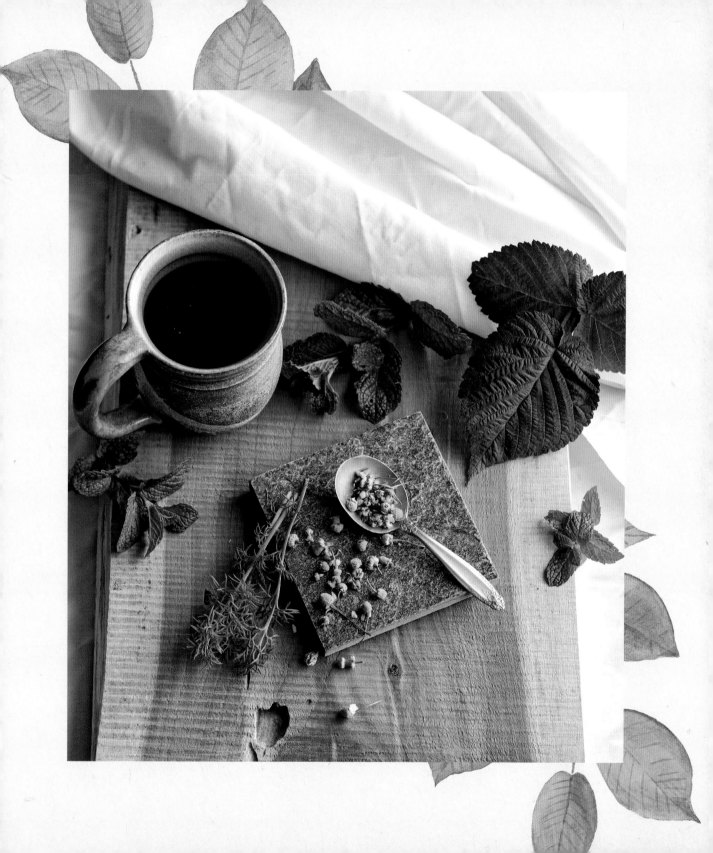

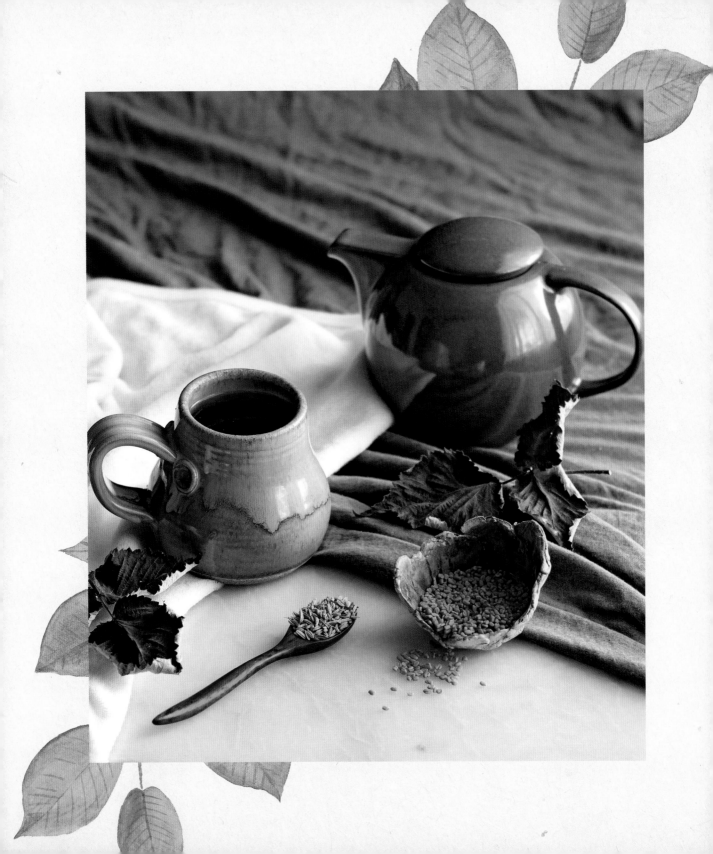

LACTATION TEA

For women who are committed to breastfeeding, it can be disheartening if their supply of breast milk drops. This tea can be very helpful to promote lactation if this happens. Fenugreek is an effective traditional remedy that has been used for centuries for increasing milk supply, and both red raspberry leaf and fennel seed also support healthy lactation. If you do experience a sudden drop in supply, please contact your local lactation consultant as soon as possible.

Yield: about 2 cups (480 ml)

Ingredients
2 cups (480 ml) water
2 tbsp (30 g) fenugreek seed
2 tbsp (2 g) dried red raspberry leaf
1 tbsp (8 g) fennel seed

Instructions
Bring the water to a boil and pour over the herbs. Let the infusion steep for 10 to 15 minutes, then strain out the herbs before drinking. For a stronger tea, follow the directions on page 15 for a long or overnight infusion. This tea can be consumed hot or iced.

Drink 1 to 2 cups (240 to 480 ml) daily to help promote lactation.

Tip: Fenugreek is a seed that has a strong maple syrup scent. If you drink this tea for a period of time, you may notice that your sweat, urine and breast milk may start to smell a bit like maple syrup.

SORE NIPPLE BUTTER

Breastfeeding is an important bond between mother and infant, but it doesn't always come easy at the beginning. Many women experience sore, painful and sometimes even cracked nipples at the beginning of their breastfeeding journey. This sore nipple butter is soothing and healing and has been formulated with ingredients that are generally regarded as safe for the baby. Please know that breastfeeding shouldn't hurt, and if you are having continued soreness and pain, you should contact your local lactation consultant for assistance. They are miracle workers!

Yield: about 12 ounces (360 ml) of butter

Ingredients

For the Infused Oil
¼ cup (5 g) dried calendula flowers
¼ cup (10 g) dried marshmallow root
½ cup (120 ml) olive oil
¼ cup (60 ml) coconut oil, melted

For the Butter
4 oz (112 g) shea butter
½ cup (120 ml) herb-infused oil

Instructions

Combine the calendula and marshmallow root with the olive and coconut oils in a half-pint (236-ml) jar. Cover the jar with a lid and shake to mix well. Put the jar in a cool, dark place to infuse for 4 to 6 weeks.

When you are ready to make the butter, strain the plant material from the oil using a fine-mesh sieve. If the coconut oil has solidified in the oil infusion, gently heat it by setting the jar in a pan of warm water to melt the oil before straining. Measure out ½ cup (120 ml) of the infused oil and set aside. Save any excess oil you may have to use topically.

Put the shea butter into a double boiler on medium heat (see tips for making your own double boiler on page 20) until it has completely melted, then promptly remove from the heat. Add the flower-infused oil to the melted shea butter and stir to combine. Pour the mixture into a medium-size mixing bowl and put in the refrigerator until it just begins to solidify, about 1 hour. Remove from the refrigerator and use a hand blender to whip the mixture for several minutes into a light and smooth butter. Scrape the nipple butter out of the bowl and into jars or tins for storage.

Immediately after nursing, pat the area dry and apply a small amount of the nipple butter to help heal dry, sore and cracked nipples.

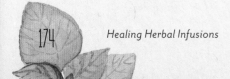

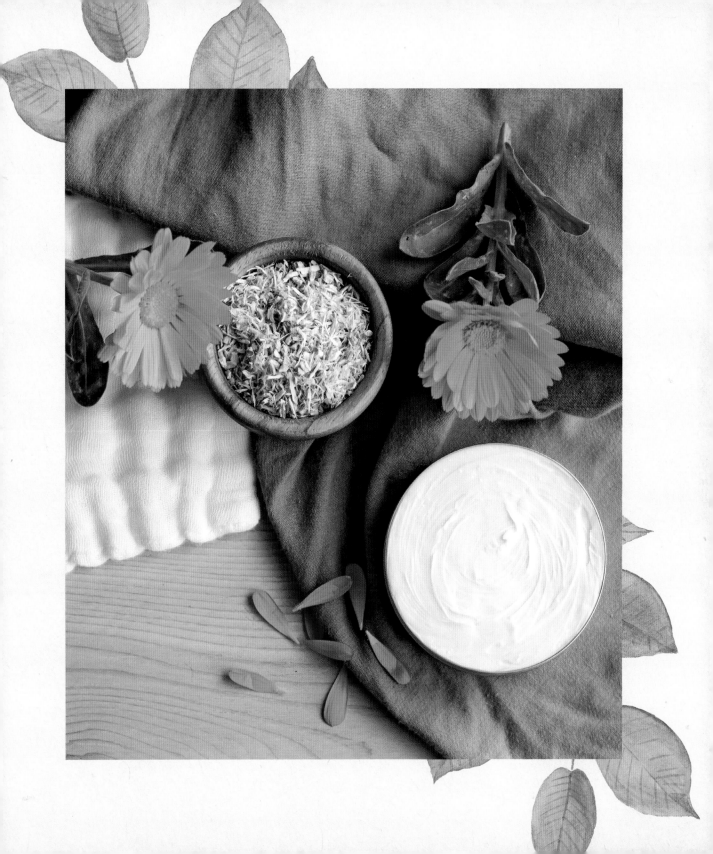

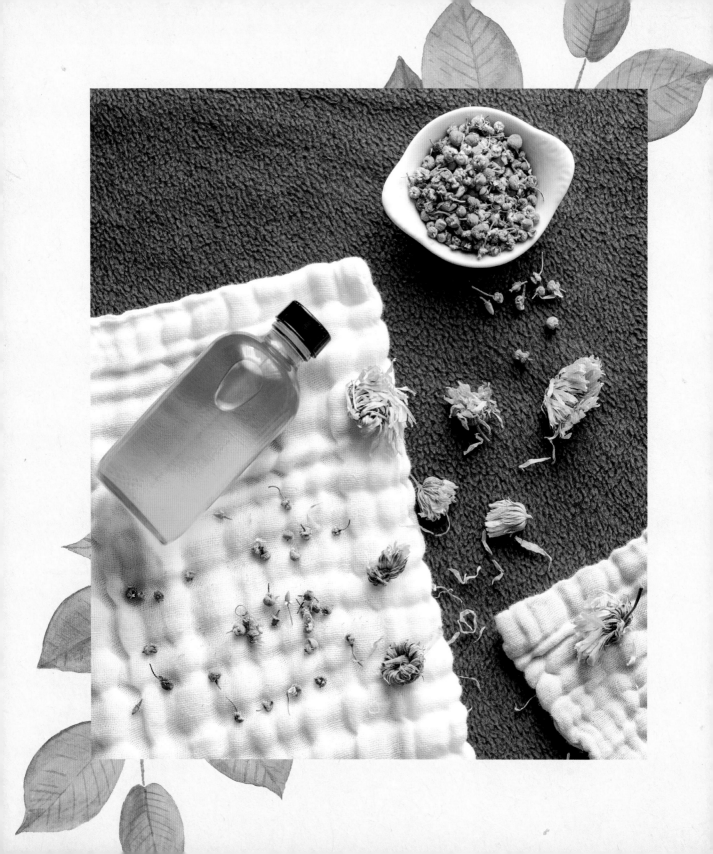

CHAMOMILE & CALENDULA BABY OIL

Baby oil is a classic item to have on hand for moisturizing sweet baby skin and for giving your little one a gentle and calming massage. This baby oil is super simple to make at home and has skin-nourishing chamomile and calendula that are perfect for sensitive skin. Sweet almond oil is not at all greasy and readily absorbs into the skin. While these ingredients rarely cause issues, I recommend doing a small patch test on your little one's hand before using to make sure there is no allergy or reaction.

Yield: about ¾ cup (180 ml)

Ingredients
¼ cup (6 g) dried chamomile flowers
¼ cup (5 g) dried calendula flowers
¾ cup (180 ml) sweet almond oil

Instructions
Combine the chamomile and calendula with the sweet almond oil in a half-pint (236-ml) jar. Cover the jar with a lid and shake to mix well. Put the jar in a cool, dark place to infuse for 4 to 6 weeks. Strain out the plant material with a fine-mesh sieve.

Apply the oil on your baby's skin as often as needed to moisturize. It is particularly nice to use after a bath and can also be used when giving your baby an infant massage.

This baby oil is safe to use on babies and children ages 3 months and older following a patch test (see page 23).

Tip: Unrefined coconut oil can be substituted for the sweet almond oil if you prefer. It will be solid at room temperature, so using the heat method on page 17 is the most effective way to infuse the flowers into the oil.

CRADLE CAP OIL

Cradle cap is a phenomenon that affects most babies at some point. Many home remedies call for rubbing a bit of coconut oil on the scalp before gently combing with a fine-tooth comb to release the dead skin. I take this a step further by adding a few herbs that will nourish the scalp and help to keep the cradle cap from returning. Calendula, violet leaves and nettle all have benefits for the skin and scalp, and are gentle enough for use on a baby. While these ingredients rarely cause issues, I recommend doing a small patch test (see page 23) on your little one's hand to make sure there is no allergy or reaction before using.

Yield: about ¾ cup (180 ml)

Ingredients
¼ cup (5 g) dried calendula flowers
2 tbsp (8 g) dried violet leaves
2 tbsp (4 g) dried nettles
½ cup (120 ml) coconut oil, melted
¼ cup (60 ml) sweet almond oil

Instructions
Combine the calendula, violet leaves and nettle with the coconut and sweet almond oils in a half-pint (236-ml) jar. Cover the jar with a lid and shake to mix well. Put the jar in a cool, dark place to infuse for 4 to 6 weeks. Strain out the plant material with a fine-mesh sieve. If the coconut oil has solidified in the oil infusion, gently heat it by setting the jar in a pan of warm water to melt the oil before straining.

Apply a small amount of the oil on the baby's scalp, then use a fine-tooth comb to release the dead skin. Use as often as needed to help remove cradle cap and to prevent it from returning.

This cradle cap oil is safe to use on babies and children ages 3 months and older following a patch test (see page 23).

Tip: This cradle cap oil is not only for babies! If you suffer from dandruff or other flaky, itchy or dry scalp conditions, try rubbing a small amount of this oil on the affected area for some relief and healing.

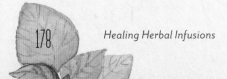

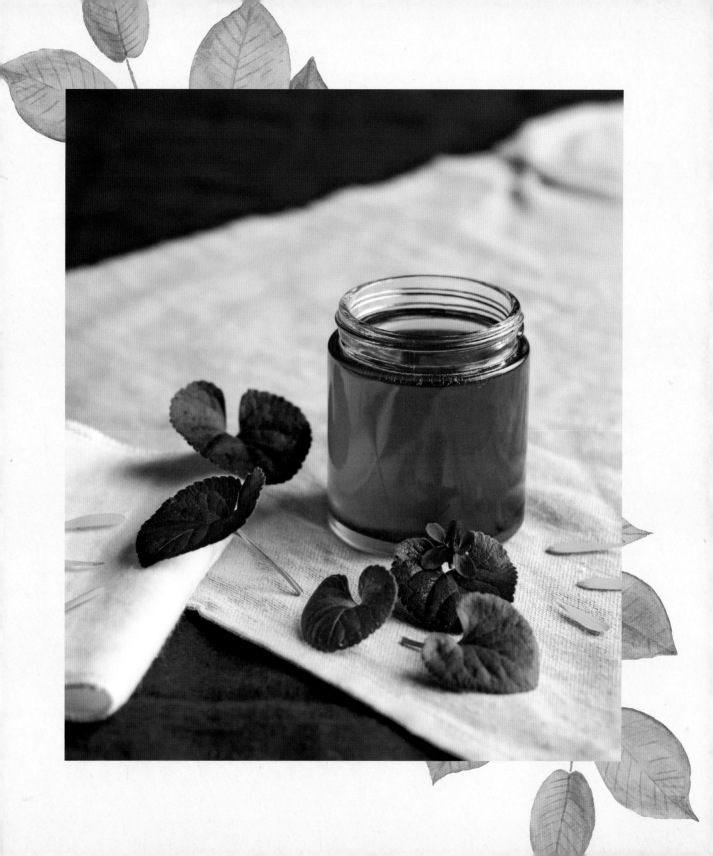

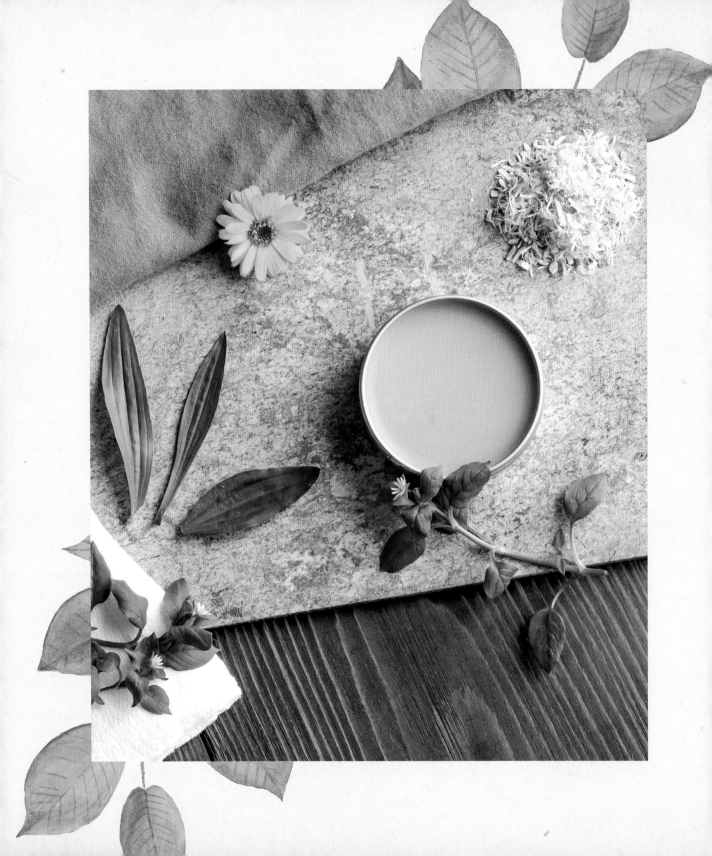

DIAPER RASH SALVE

When your little one is suffering from diaper rash, reach for this amazing salve. This is one of my most popular recipes for good reason—it works miracles! It will often clear or greatly reduce a diaper rash overnight. While the herbs in this recipe are extremely healing for a persistent and irritating rash, a big part of what makes this salve work is the large portion of beeswax, which provides a strong barrier. Use it as a preventative and you'll hardly ever have to deal with diaper rash again! While these ingredients rarely cause issues, I recommend doing a small patch test (see page 23) on your little one's hand before using to make sure there is no allergy or reaction.

Yield: about 5 ounces (150 ml) of salve

Ingredients

For the Infused Oil
2 tbsp (5 g) dried marshmallow root
2 tbsp (5 g) dried plantain leaf
2 tbsp (4 g) dried chickweed
2 tbsp (3 g) dried calendula flowers
½ cup (120 ml) coconut oil, melted
¼ cup (60 ml) sweet almond oil

For the Salve
½ cup (120 ml) infused oil
1 oz (28 g) beeswax
½ oz (14 g) shea butter

Instructions

Combine the marshmallow root, plantain, chickweed and calendula with the coconut and sweet almond oils in a half-pint (236-ml) jar. Cover the jar with a lid and shake to mix well. Put the jar in a cool, dark place to infuse for 4 to 6 weeks.

When you are ready to make the salve, strain the herbs from the oil using a fine-mesh sieve. If the coconut oil has solidified in the oil infusion, gently heat it by setting the jar in a pan of warm water to melt the oil before straining. Measure out ½ cup (120 ml) of the infused oil, saving any excess oil for later use if you wish. Put the oil into a double boiler on medium heat (see tips for making your own double boiler on page 20). Add the beeswax to the oil and continue to heat until it has completely melted. Next, add the shea butter, and when it has melted, remove the mixture from the heat. Carefully pour the mixture into jars or tins. Let the salve cool and set up for 3 to 4 hours before use.

Apply as often as needed to help heal and prevent diaper rash.

This diaper rash salve is safe to use on babies and children ages 3 months and older following a patch test (see page 23).

BOO-BOO BALM

For life's little boo-boos, this balm can make it better! Sometimes the power of suggestion and the ritual of applying a balm to an "owie" is all that is needed for little ones, but the great part about this boo-boo balm is that it truly has amazing healing benefits. It has the gentle strength of calendula, lavender and chamomile flowers, all of which speed healing. Use this balm on minor cuts, scrapes, bruises, bug bites, rashes and dry skin for quick relief.

Yield: about 5 ounces (150 ml) of balm

Ingredients

For the Infused Oil
¼ cup (5 g) dried calendula flowers

2 tbsp (5 g) dried lavender flowers

2 tbsp (3 g) dried chamomile flowers

½ cup (120 ml) coconut oil, melted

¼ cup (60 ml) sweet almond oil

For the Balm
½ cup (120 ml) infused oil

½ oz (14 g) beeswax

½ oz (14 g) shea butter

Instructions

Combine the calendula, lavender and chamomile with the coconut and sweet almond oils in a half-pint (236-ml) jar. Cover the jar with a lid and shake to mix well. Put the jar in a cool, dark place to infuse for 4 to 6 weeks.

When you are ready to make the balm, strain the herbs from the oil using a fine-mesh sieve. If the coconut oil has solidified in the oil infusion, gently heat it by setting the jar in a pan of warm water to melt the oil before straining. Measure out ½ cup (120 ml) of the infused oil, saving any excess oil for later use if you wish. Put the oil into a double boiler on medium heat (see tips for making your own double boiler on page 20). Add the beeswax to the oil and continue to heat until it has completely melted. Next, add the shea butter, and when it has melted, remove the mixture from the heat. Carefully pour the mixture into jars or tins. Let the balm cool and set up for 3 to 4 hours before use.

Apply as often as needed to help gently heal minor cuts, scrapes, bruises, bug bites, rashes and dry skin.

This boo-boo balm is safe to use on babies and children ages 6 months and older following a patch test (see page 23).

Tip: Beyond boo-boos, this salve can really do it all! It works well as an all-purpose ointment for almost any minor skin ailment, and it is one I recommend always having on hand.

Healing Herbal Infusions

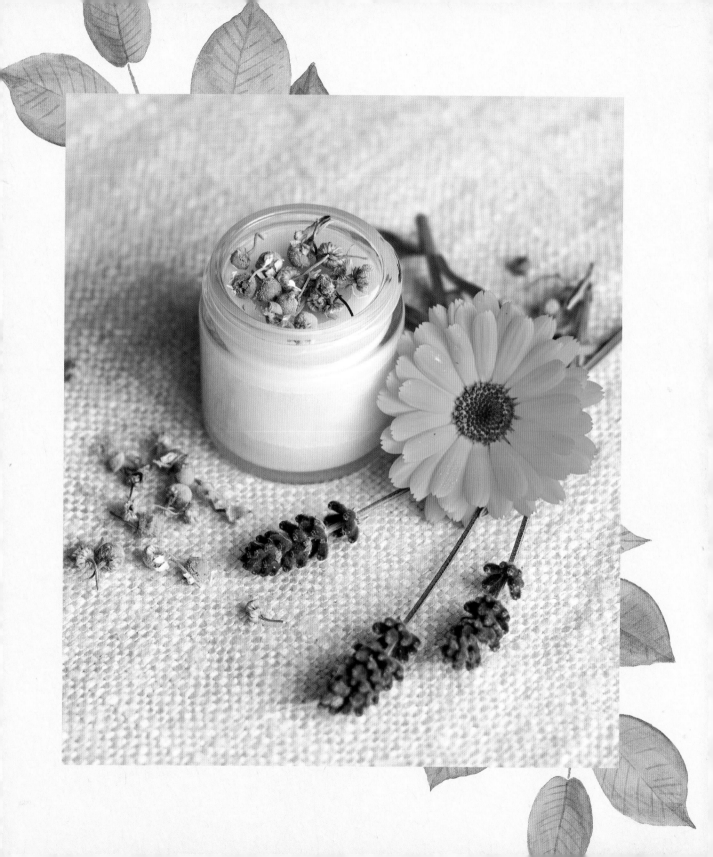

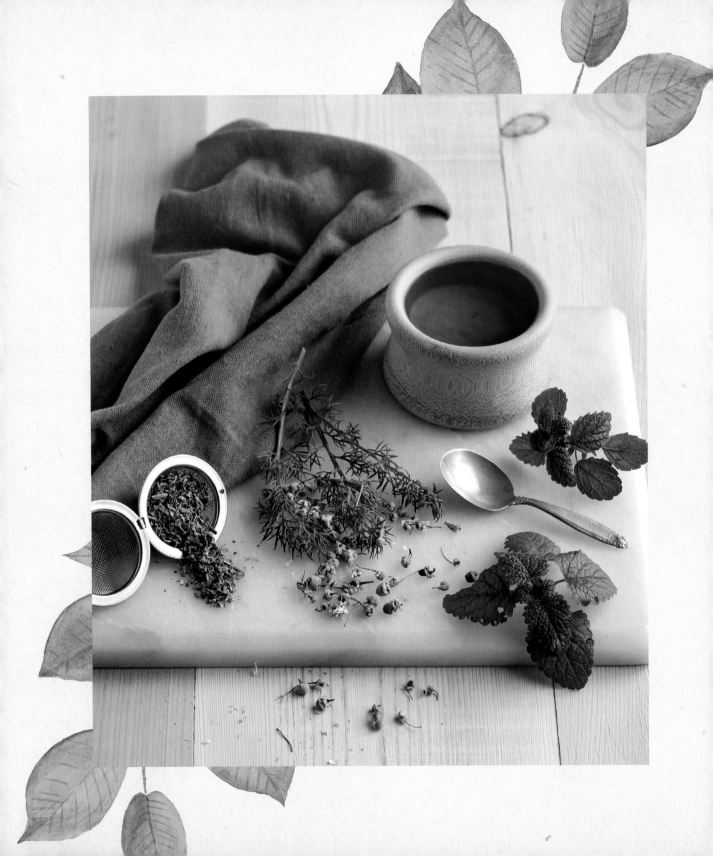

CHILDREN'S CALMING TEA

It's a well-known fact that children can easily become overstimulated and, for lack of a better word, rambunctious. When it comes time to bring a child back to his or her center, this calming tea can really help. Catnip in particular is an amazing herbal ally for children, as it has a gentle calming effect that promotes relaxation and sleep. Lemon balm and chamomile are flavorful herbs that are safe for children and also have a calming effect. All three of these herbs have the added benefit of being good for children's digestion. In the summertime, pour this tea into small popsicle molds for a fun, healthy and relaxing treat. Small amounts of this tea can be given to teething babies over the age of 6 months for some relief.

Yield: about 2 cups (480 ml)

Ingredients
2 cups (480 ml) water
2 tbsp (3 g) dried chamomile flowers
1 tbsp (1 g) dried lemon balm
1 tbsp (1 g) dried catnip
1–2 tbsp (15–30 ml) honey (optional— not to be given to babies under the age of 1)

Instructions
Bring the water to a boil and pour over the herbs. Let the infusion steep for 10 to 15 minutes, then strain out the herbs and stir in the honey (if using) before drinking. This tea can be consumed hot or iced.

This tea is safe for babies and children ages 6 months and older. I recommend doing a patch test (see page 23) by rubbing a little bit of the tea on the back of the hand or inner arm to see if there is any reaction before consuming, especially with younger babies and children.

Have the child drink 1 to 2 times per day for a calming and centering effect. Follow these dosage guidelines by age:

6 months to 1 year: 1 to 2 teaspoons (5 to 10 ml) total daily

1 to 2 years: 2 to 4 teaspoons (10 to 20 ml) total daily

3 to 7 years: 2 to 4 tablespoons (30 to 60 ml) total daily

8 to 12 years: ¼ to ½ cup (60 to 120 ml) total daily

13 and over: 1 to 2 cups (240 to 480 ml) total daily

ELDERBERRY & ECHINACEA GLYCERITE FOR COLDS & FLUS

Glycerites are similar to tinctures, but instead of being made with alcohol, they are made with a sweet vegetable glycerine. This makes them perfect for use with children or whenever alcohol is best to be avoided. Elderberry and echinacea are powerful immune system herbs that are safe for children to take during times of illness to promote wellness and a faster recovery.

Yield: about 1⅓ cups (320 ml)

Ingredients
¼ cup (30 g) dried elderberries
¼ cup (20 g) dried echinacea root
1 cup (240 ml) vegetable glycerine
⅓ cup (80 ml) water

Instructions
Combine the elderberries, echinacea, glycerine and water in a pint-size (473-ml) jar. Cover the jar with a lid and shake to mix well. Put the jar in a cool, dark place to infuse for 4 to 6 weeks. Strain out the herbs using a fine-mesh sieve. Store the glycerite in small bottles with droppers for easy use.

This glycerite is safe to use on babies and children ages 1 year and older. I recommend doing a patch test (see page 23) by rubbing a little bit of the glycerite on the back of the hand or inner arm to see if there is any reaction before consuming, especially with younger babies and children.

Have the child take 2 to 3 times per day at the first sign of a cold or flu for the most benefit. It can be taken straight or mixed into water or tea if you prefer. Please follow these dosage guidelines by age:

1 to 2 years: 5 to 8 drops total daily

3 to 7 years: 8 to 15 drops total daily

8 to 12 years: 15 to 30 drops total daily

13 and over: 3 teaspoons (15 ml) total daily

Tip: If you have access to fresh black elderberries, they can be substituted in this recipe. Use ½ cup (60 g) of the fresh berries in place of dried.

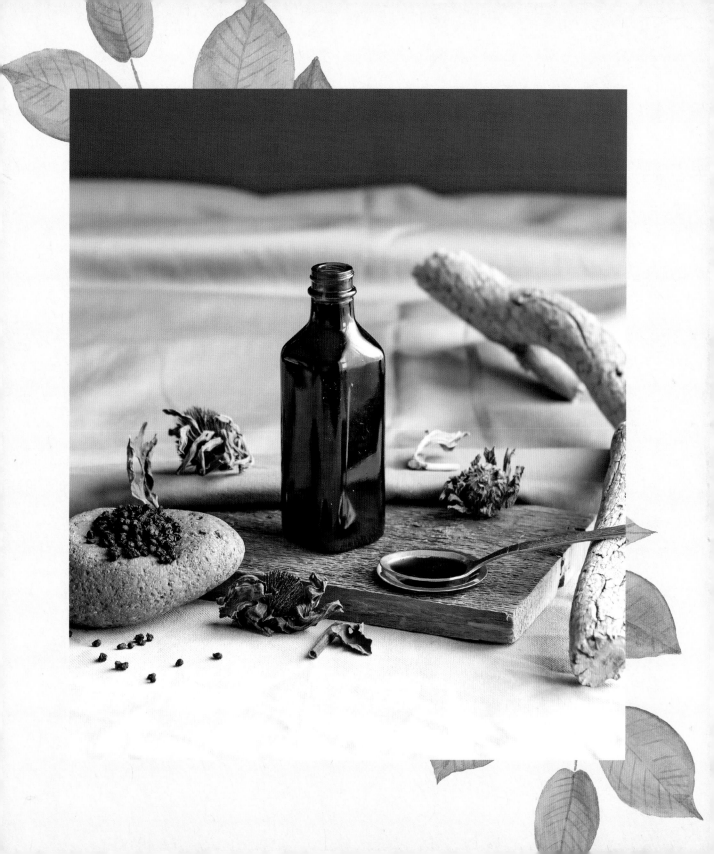

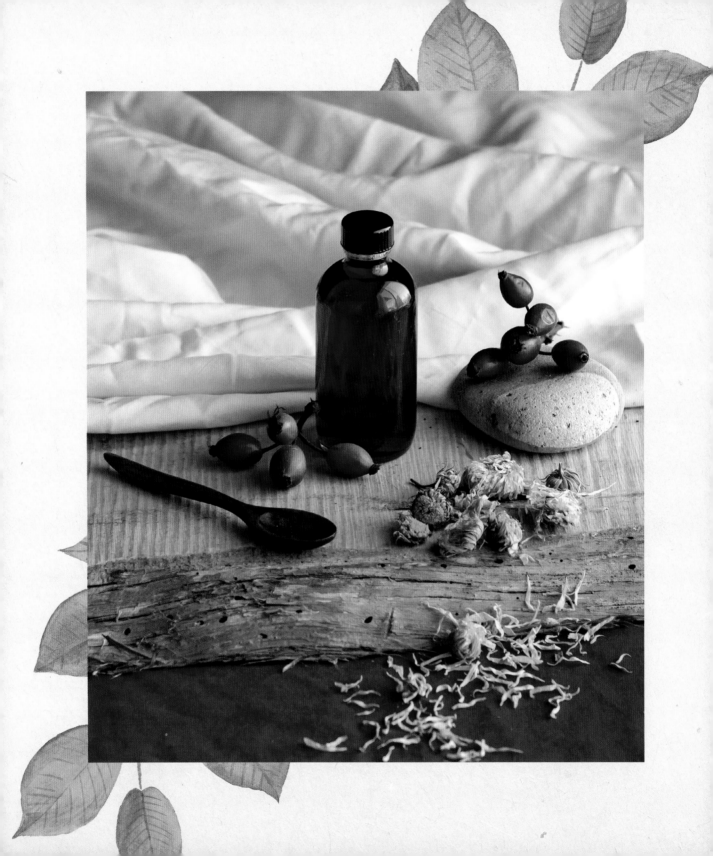

CALENDULA & ROSE HIP IMMUNE-BOOSTING GLYCERITE

While calendula is well known for its external skin benefits, it can also safely be used internally as an antimicrobial immune booster. Rose hips are extremely high in vitamin C, which helps to promote immune function. When used in combination, these two herbs boost the immune system and help to shorten the duration of colds and flus. This glycerite is safe for children, and it is the perfect choice for anyone who wishes to avoid tinctures made from alcohol.

Yield: about 1⅓ cups (320 ml)

Ingredients
½ cup (6 g) dried calendula flowers
¼ cup (30 g) dried rose hips
1 cup (240 ml) vegetable glycerine
⅓ cup (80 ml) water

Instructions
Combine the calendula, rose hips, glycerine and water in a pint-size (473-ml) jar. Cover the jar with a lid and shake to mix well. Put the jar in a cool, dark place to infuse for 4 to 6 weeks. Strain out the herbs using a fine-mesh sieve. Store the glycerite in small bottles with droppers for easy use.

This glycerite is safe to use on babies and children ages 1 year and older. I recommend doing a patch test (see page 23) by rubbing a little bit of the glycerite on the back of the hand or inner arm to see if there is any reaction before consuming, especially with younger babies and children.

Have the child take 2 to 3 times per day to support the immune system and to prevent illness. It can be taken straight or mixed into water or tea if you prefer. Please follow these dosing guidelines by age:

1 to 2 years: 5 to 8 drops total daily

3 to 7 years: 8 to 15 drops total daily

8 to 12 years: 15 to 30 drops total daily

13 and over: 3 teaspoons (15 ml) total daily

Tip: If you have access to fresh calendula flowers and rose hips, they can be substituted in this recipe. Use 1 cup (12 g) fresh calendula flowers and ½ cup (60 g) fresh rose hips in place of dried.

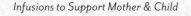

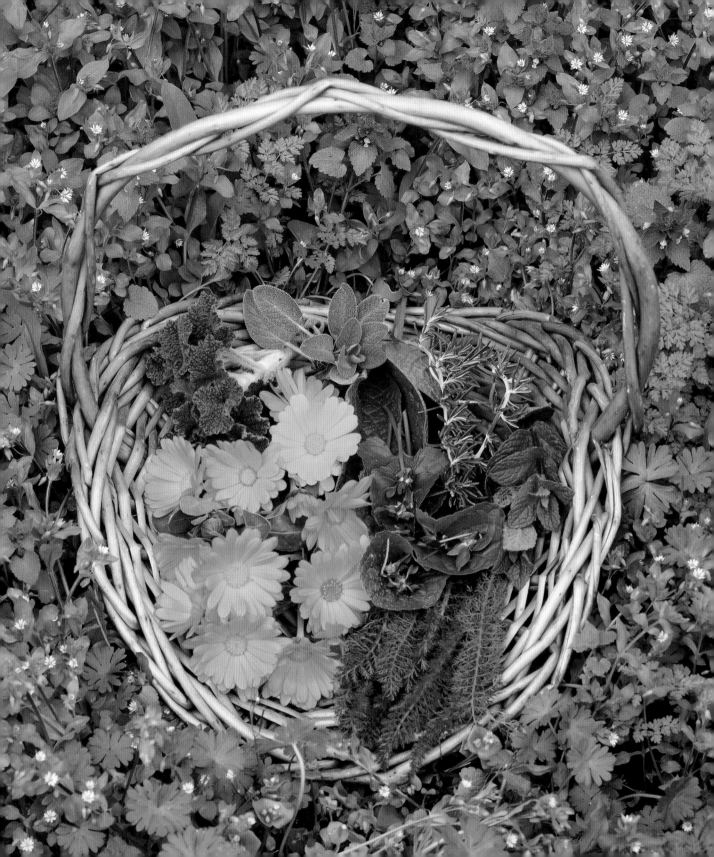

HERB & FLOWER PROFILES

The following is a list of every herb that is used in the recipes in this book and a brief description of their benefits and herbal actions, plus a few other notes of interest. This is a great starting point to read about the specifics of each herb, and it will help you begin or continue your journey in herbal medicine. For further reading on herbs and their actions, check out the books I list in the resources section on page 200.

Arnica (Arnica montana): This sunny yellow flower is in the sunflower family. It is anti-inflammatory and an anesthetic pain reliever. It is best used topically in creams, salves and ointments to help reduce pain and inflammation from sore muscles, joints, strains, sprains and bruises. Do not use internally, as it is toxic if consumed in large amounts. Use arnica in Arnica Salve for Sprains & Bruises (page 49).

Astragalus (Astragalus membranaceus): The root of a legume family plant, astragalus is commonly used in Traditional Chinese Medicine. It is an adaptogen, helping protect the body from physical, mental or emotional stress. It is also an energy tonic and immune booster, and it has antiviral, antibacterial, anti-inflammatory and diuretic properties. Use astragalus in Elderberry & Astragalus Tincture (page 31) and Liver Support Tonic (page 93).

Basil (Ocimum basilicum): This common kitchen herb is also highly medicinal. Basil is a carminative digestive aid and a pain-relieving anti-inflammatory. It is also antibacterial, antioxidant and antispasmodic. As an emmenagogue, it should not be used in large amounts during pregnancy; small culinary amounts are fine. Use basil in Fresh Kitchen Herb Oxymel (page 40) and Basil, Thyme & Oregano Tea for Chronic Pain (page 58).

Birch Bark (Betula spp.): The inner bark of the birch tree is a powerful analgesic painkiller. It is also anti-inflammatory, astringent, aromatic, and as a febrifuge it assists the body to reduce fever. Only forage for birch bark from dead and dying trees, as taking from live trees can damage them. Use birch bark in White Willow & Birch Bark Tea for Pain Relief (page 57).

Blackberry Leaf (Rubus fruticosus): The leaf of blackberry brambles is high in vitamins, antioxidants and flavonoids. Due to its high tannin content, blackberry leaf is very astringent and can help to heal mouth sores, sore throats, ulcers, hemorrhoids and diarrhea. It also makes a highly effective face wash. Use blackberry leaf in Witch Hazel & Blackberry Leaf Face Wash (page 156).

Black Pepper (Piper nigrum): A common kitchen spice, black pepper is antioxidant, antispasmodic, diuretic, aromatic and a warming stimulant that improves circulation. The piperine in black pepper makes the curcumin in turmeric more bioavailable. Use black pepper in Turmeric & Black Pepper Tea for Chronic Inflammation (page 61) and Roasted Chicory Root Chai (page 111).

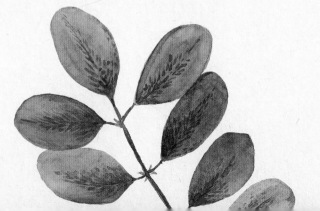

Burdock Root (Arctium lappa): The long taproot of the burdock thistle is a popular food in Asian cultures. It is antibacterial and antifungal, and as a hepatic it strengthens and tones the liver. It is also commonly used as a bitter digestive aid. The burrs on the burdock plant were the original inspiration for Velcro. Use burdock in Prebiotic Honey Electuary (page 104) and Dandelion & Burdock Root Bitters (page 115).

Calendula (Calendula officinalis): This beautiful orange or yellow flower is vulnerary, promoting the healing of wounds. It is also antiseptic, antimicrobial, antifungal, anti-inflammatory and good for the lymphatic system. Calendula is excellent used topically in creams, salves or ointments for all skin irritations, scars and bruises, or internally as a tea for fevers, ulcers, cramps, indigestion, diarrhea and swollen glands. It can be used by the whole family, and it is even mild enough for babies and young children. Use calendula in Four-Herb Wound Salve (page 62), Herbal Honey Burn Ointment (page 65), Sunburn Aloe Infusion (page 69), Eczema Relief Salve (page 97), Calming Massage Oil (page 128), Healing Flower-Whipped Body Butter (page 143), Cocoa Mint Cracked Heel Balm (page 151), Blemish Balm (page 155), Sore Nipple Butter (page 174), Chamomile & Calendula Baby Oil (page 177), Cradle Cap Oil (page 178), Diaper Rash Salve (page 181), Boo-Boo Balm (page 182) and Calendula & Rose Hip Immune-Boosting Glycerite (page 189).

California Poppy (Eschscholzia californica): The state flower of California, it is native to western United States and northwest Mexico. California poppy is sedative, analgesic, antispasmodic and it can be used externally as an antimicrobial. It is a common myth that it is illegal to pick these flowers in the state of California; they are only protected on government property, but are free to forage everywhere else. Use it in California Poppy Tincture for Relaxation (page 132).

Cannabis (Cannabis sativa subsp.): This controversial plant is becoming more popular for medicinal use as it becomes legal in an increasing number of places. Cannabis is analgesic, antispasmodic, nervine, psychedelic and sedative. Tetrahydrocannabinol (THC) and cannabidiol (CBD) are the main medicinal compounds in cannabis, but there are many others. THC has the most psychoactivity ("stoned" feeling), while CBD is pain relieving with minimal psychoactivity. Please check all of your local laws and requirements for legal use before using cannabis as medicine. Use it in Cannabis-Infused Coconut Oil for Body Aches (page 50).

Cardamom (Eletteria cardamomum): This quintessential chai spice in the ginger family has many medicinal benefits. Cardamom is a powerful carminative digestive aid that is aromatic and warming. It is also analgesic, antispasmodic, diuretic and even may have some anticancer properties. Use cardamom in Fennel & Cardamom After-Meal Tummy Tea (page 107) and Roasted Chicory Root Chai (page 111).

Catnip (Nepeta cataria): Not just for our feline friends, this mint-family herb is excellent for children and adults alike. Catnip is a soothing and mild sedative and is antispasmodic. As a diaphoretic, it induces perspiration and is an effective fever reducer. It is also an anti-inflammatory pain reliever and is good for digestive issues. Use catnip in Fever-Reducing Tea (page 85), Four-Mints Herbal Hot or Iced Tea (page 112), Sleep Well Tea (page 124) and Children's Calming Tea (page 185).

Cayenne (Caspicum minimum): This spicy pepper is a warming circulatory stimulant and a powerful pain reliever when used topically. Cayenne is also a carminative digestive aid, immune booster, heart tonic and has antimicrobial properties. Use cayenne in Immune-Boosting Vinegar Infusion (Hot or Not) (page 43) and Saint John's Wort & Cayenne Warming Oil (page 53).

Chamomile (Matricaria recutita): A small flower in the daisy family, chamomile is best known for its sleep-promoting properties. It is a nervine herb, as it calms the nervous system and helps the mind and body to relax. Chamomile is also a strong anti-inflammatory pain reliever and a carminative digestive aid. It is a very safe herb that can be used for children and babies. Those with ragweed allergies should avoid using chamomile. Use chamomile in Headache Relief Tea (page 73), Sleep Well Tea (page 124), Calming Massage Oil (page 128), Rejuvenating Flower Bath Soak (page 136), Chamomile, Marshmallow & Vanilla Chapped Lip Balm (page 152), Blemish Balm (page 155), Pregnancy Tonic Tea (page 170), Chamomile & Calendula Baby Oil (page 177), Boo-Boo Balm (page 182) and Children's Calming Tea (page 185).

Chicory Root (Cichorium intybus): The root of the chicory plant is a bitter digestive aid that is high in inulin, a prebiotic compound that boosts the amount of probiotics in the gut. It is soothing, calming and anti-inflammatory. Roasted chicory root tastes surprisingly like coffee when made into a tea, but without any caffeine. Use chicory root in Prebiotic Honey Electuary (page 104) and Roasted Chicory Root Chai (page 111).

Chickweed (Stellaria media): A low-growing, early spring plant that can be found nearly everywhere, chickweed is mucilaginous and a hydrating emollient that is excellent for skin conditions. It is cooling, astringent and an anti-inflammatory wound healer. Chickweed is also a very nutritious wild green that can be used as food as well as medicine. Use chickweed in Sunburn Aloe Infusion (page 69), Eczema Relief Salve (page 97), Soothing Chickweed Lotion Bars (page 147), Dry Hands Balm (page 148) and Diaper Rash Salve (page 181).

Cinnamon (Cinnamomum verum): This common aromatic kitchen spice is warming, improves digestion and may help to lower blood sugar. Cinnamon has powerful antibacterial, antiviral and antifungal properties, making it very beneficial for the immune system. Its pleasant flavor improves the taste of many medicinal preparations. Use cinnamon in Vitamin C Tea (page 28), Elderberry, Ginger & Cinnamon Honey (page 39), Horehound Sore Throat Syrup (page 78), Fever-Reducing Tea (page 85), Ginger & Turmeric Decoction & Honey Syrup (page 103), Marshmallow & Cinnamon Digestive Tea (page 108), Roasted Chicory Root Chai (page 111) and Sarsaparilla & Fennel Bitters (page 116).

Cloves (Syzygium aromaticum): Like cinnamon, cloves are another common warming and aromatic kitchen spice. They are a highly effective analgesic pain reliever and are well known for greatly reducing tooth pain. They are also anti-inflammatory, antiseptic, antibacterial, astringent and a digestive aid. Use cloves in Clove Whiskey Tincture for Tooth Pain (page 89) and Roasted Chicory Root Chai (page 111).

Comfrey (Symphytum officinale): A potent anti-inflammatory wound healer, both the root and leaves can be used. Also known as knitbone, comfrey is commonly used externally as a poultice for wounds, sores, burns and fractures. It speeds healing and promotes the growth of new skin cells. It should not be used on deep or infected wounds as it will heal the surface first and could potentially seal in an infection. There is conflicting evidence on the safety of using comfrey internally, so proceed with caution. Use comfrey in Four-Herb Wound Salve (page 62) and Herbal Honey Burn Ointment (page 65).

Dandelion Root (Taraxacum officinale): The root of the common dandelion is a powerful liver detoxifier, blood purifier and diuretic. It also encourages digestion and helps to calm an upset stomach. It is high in antioxidants and may be beneficial for regulating cholesterol levels. Roasted dandelion root makes a wonderful tea that tastes similar to coffee. Use dandelion root in Liver Support Tonic (page 93), Prebiotic Honey Electuary (page 104), Dandelion & Burdock Root Bitters (page 115) and Long Infusion Fertility Tea (page 169).

Echinacea (Echinacea angustifolia): Also known as coneflower, echinacea is a strong but safe immune stimulant that is most effective when taken at the earliest sign of illness or infection. It also has powerful antimicrobial, antifungal and antibacterial properties. It is particularly good at healing respiratory infections and sore throats. Use echinacea in Super Immunity Infusion Tea (page 27), Echinacea Root & Flower Tincture (page 32) and Elderberry & Echinacea Glycerite for Colds & Flus (page 186).

Elder (Sambucus nigra): Both the flowers and the berries of the elder tree are highly medicinal, particularly for colds and flus. The flowers induce sweating to lower fever and are also beneficial for skin conditions. The berries are a super potent antiviral and an immune system booster. Due to its powerful ability to invoke an immune system response, elder should not be used by those with any type of autoimmune disease. Use elderflowers in Fever-Reducing Tea (page 85) and Healing Flower-Whipped Body Butter (page 143). Use elderberries in Super Immunity Infusion Tea (page 27), Elderberry & Astragalus Tincture (page 31), Elderberry, Ginger & Cinnamon Honey (page 39) and Elderberry & Echinacea Glycerite for Colds & Flus (page 186).

Fennel (Foeniculum vulgare): The seeds from the fennel bulb are highly beneficial for the digestive system. They stimulate digestion and appetite, and also help with indigestion. Fennel seeds are antispasmodic, anti-inflammatory and as a galactagogue they increase production of breastmilk. Use fennel seeds in Fennel & Cardamom After-Meal Tummy Tea (page 107), Sarsaparilla & Fennel Bitters (page 116) and Lactation Tea (page 173).

Feverfew (Tanacetum parthenium): This flower in the daisy family is a potent anti-inflammatory that is excellent for relieving headaches and preventing migraines. It has also been known to alleviate the pain and swelling from rheumatoid arthritis. Feverfew should be avoided by pregnant women and those with ragweed allergies. Use it in Feverfew Migraine Preventative Tincture (page 74).

Garlic (Allium sativum): Possibly the most important herb for boosting the immune system and for preventing colds and flus. Raw garlic has super powerful antibacterial, antimicrobial and antiseptic properties, making it excellent for treating infections. It is also highly effective at improving circulation, lowering blood sugar and maintaining healthy cholesterol levels. A clove of garlic a day keeps the doctor away! Use garlic in Fermented Garlic, Ginger & Sage in Honey (page 35) and Immune-Boosting Vinegar Infusion (Hot or Not) (page 43).

Ginger (Zingiber officinale): This root is a warming immune system stimulant that also increases circulation, relieves nausea and intestinal pain and is an antispasmodic for digestion. Ginger is also beneficial for helping to sweat out a fever, and it has powerful anti-inflammatory and antimicrobial properties. Use ginger in Super Immunity Infusion Tea (page 27), Fermented Garlic, Ginger & Sage in Honey (page

35), Elderberry, Ginger & Cinnamon Honey (page 39), Immune-Boosting Vinegar Infusion (Hot or Not) (page 43), Sage, Marshmallow & Ginger Sore Throat Tea (page 77), Ginger & Turmeric Decoction & Honey Syrup (page 103), Roasted Chicory Root Chai (page 111) and Herbal Vinegar Infusion for Heartburn (page 119).

Hawthorn Berries (Crataegus monogyna):
The berries from the hawthorn tree are an effective heart tonic that can help treat high or low blood pressure and heart disease. They are also astringent and a diuretic and can help to regulate cholesterol levels. Beyond physical heart issues, hawthorn berries can also help to heal the emotions from a broken heart. Please consult with your doctor before using hawthorn berries if you have heart conditions or if you are on any kind of medication for the heart or blood pressure. Use hawthorn berries in Hawthorn & Hibiscus Tea for the Heart (page 90).

Hibiscus (Hibiscus sabdariffa):
This beautiful tropical flower is antibacterial, astringent and high in antioxidants and vitamin C. Hibiscus is also highly effective at reducing blood pressure. Pregnant women should avoid using hibiscus. If you are taking blood pressure medication, please consult your doctor before using hibiscus. Use hibiscus in Vitamin C Tea (page 28), Hawthorn & Hibiscus Tea for the Heart (page 90) and Long Infusion Fertility Tea (page 169).

Holy Basil (Ocimum sanctum):
Also known as tulsi, this aromatic relative of culinary basil is a powerful adaptogen that is one of the best herbs for reducing stress and anxiety. Holy basil is also high in antioxidants and has antibacterial, antifungal and anti-inflammatory properties. Use holy basil in De-Stress Tea (page 127).

Horehound (Marrubium vulgare):
This astringent and highly bitter herb has become widely naturalized in many places, making it generally easy to forage for. Horehound has been used as folk medicine for respiratory ailments and sore throats for centuries. It is an effective expectorant and is anti-inflammatory. Use it in Horehound Sore Throat Syrup (page 78).

Juniper Berries (Juniperus communis):
The berries from the juniper tree have many medicinal properties, including being a powerful diuretic, making them beneficial for the kidneys and urinary tract. They are also astringent, antiseptic and antiviral. Consult a guidebook when foraging juniper berries, as some varieties are mildly toxic and should be avoided. Use juniper berries in UTI Relief Tea (page 94).

Lavender (Lavendula spp.):
This aromatic purple flower is a common landscaping plant. Lavender is calming, helps to relieve tension and stress and is a natural antidepressant. It is also antibacterial, antifungal, antiseptic and antispasmodic. Due to its pleasing scent and anti-inflammatory properties, it is often used in skin care products. Use lavender in Lavender & Peppermint Sore Muscle Oil (page 54), Herbal Honey Burn Ointment (page 65), Calming Massage Oil (page 128), Rejuvenating Flower Bath Soak (page 136), Relaxing Herbal Face Steam (page 139), Healing Flower-Whipped Body Butter (page 143), Dry Hands Balm (page 148), Blemish Balm (page 155) and Boo-Boo Balm (page 182).

Lemon Balm (Melissa officinalis):
A mint-family herb with a distinct and highly aromatic lemony scent, lemon balm is calming for the nervous and digestive system due to its volatile oils and antispasmodic properties. It is an effective remedy for depression,

(continued)

anxiety, stress and insomnia. It is also a powerful antiviral that is commonly used to relieve cold sores caused by the herpes virus. Lemon balm is safe and highly regarded for children, and is often used to calm a sleepless or hyperactive child. Use lemon balm in Headache Relief Tea (page 73), Lemon Balm Cold Sore Balm (page 98), Four-Mints Herbal Hot or Iced Tea (page 112) and Children's Calming Tea (page 185).

Marshmallow (Althaea officinalis): The root of the marshmallow plant is a highly mucilaginous and emollient tonic. It is anti-inflammatory, soothing to the throat, stomach and digestive tract and is beneficial for bladder and kidney infections. Marshmallow root is also used externally for moisturizing dry and chapped skin. Use marshmallow root in Sage, Marshmallow & Ginger Sore Throat Tea (page 77), UTI Relief Tea (page 94), Prebiotic Honey Electuary (page 104), Marshmallow & Cinnamon Digestive Tea (page 108), Cocoa Mint Cracked Heel Balm (page 151), Chamomile, Marshmallow & Vanilla Chapped Lip Balm (page 152), Sore Nipple Butter (page 174) and Diaper Rash Salve (page 181).

Mullein (Verbascum thapsus): This widespread "weed" commonly grows along roadsides and in disturbed areas, and it is easily distinguished by its tall yellow flower spike. Mullein leaf is antispasmodic and a powerful expectorant, making it beneficial for the respiratory system. The flowers are antiseptic and anti-inflammatory, and they are often used as an effective treatment for ear infections. Use mullein flowers in Mullein Flower Earache Oil (page 86).

Nettle (Urtica dioica): This springtime plant grows wild in many places, but has a painful sting when fresh, so care should be taken when harvesting. The stinging compound is removed when the herb is dried or heated. Nettle is a powerful detoxifier and tonic herb that strengthens the urinary, digestive, respiratory and reproductive systems. It is high in many vitamins and minerals, and it makes a highly nutritive tonic tea. It is also beneficial for the hair and scalp. Use nettle in Liver Support Tonic (page 93), Nettle & Oatstraw Long-Infused Tea for Vitality (page 123), Spruce & Nettle Beard Oil (page 164), Long Infusion Fertility Tea (page 169) and Cradle Cap Oil (page 178).

Oatstraw (Avena sativa): The oat grass stem of common oats has immense medicinal benefits. As a nervine, it helps to calm the nerves and to reduce stress and anxiety. Oatstraw is also very high in vitamins, minerals and trace nutrients. It is most commonly consumed as a strong tea and can be taken on a daily basis. It is an extremely safe herb that can be taken by the entire family. Oat tops can be used in place of oatstraw. Use oatstraw in Nettle & Oatstraw Long-Infused Tea for Vitality (page 123).

Onion (Allium cepa): A kitchen staple for culinary use, onions also have medicinal benefits. They are an immune system powerhouse with antibacterial, antiviral, antimicrobial, antifungal and anti-inflammatory properties. They are also high in antioxidants, flavonoids and many vitamins and minerals. Use onion in Fermented Red Onion & Thyme in Honey (page 36).

Oregano (Origanum vulgare): This common perennial culinary herb is also great for the immune system with antibacterial, antiviral and antiseptic properties. It also has powerful anti-inflammatory benefits, and it can be used internally or topically to reduce pain or boost the immune system. Use oregano in Fresh Kitchen Herb Oxymel (page 40), Immune-Boosting Vinegar Infusion (Hot or Not) (page 43), Oregano-Infused Oil with Lemon (page 44) and Basil, Thyme & Oregano Tea for Chronic Pain (page 58).

Passionflower (Passiflora incarnata): This vining plant has beautiful flowers that have been traditionally used as medicine for centuries. Passionflower is a sedative and can help to treat insomnia and other sleep issues. It is also antispasmodic, and it is effective at treating anxiety and relaxing the mind and body. Passionflower should not be used by pregnant women. Use passionflower in De-Stress Tea (page 127) and Passionflower-Infused Wine (page 135).

Peppermint (Mentha piperita): This classic mint-family plant is easy to grow and can sometimes become invasive. As a cooling carminative and antispasmodic, it is especially good for the digestive system, helping to treat nausea, indigestion, flatulence, acid reflux and bad breath. It is also a powerful antimicrobial and pain reliever. Lactating women should avoid using peppermint as it can dry up your supply. Use peppermint in Lavender & Peppermint Sore Muscle Oil (page 54), Thyme, Peppermint & Honey Tea for Coughs (page 81), Four-Mints Herbal Hot or Iced Tea (page 112), Herbal Vinegar Infusion for Heartburn (page 119), Relaxing Herbal Face Steam (page 139) and Pregnancy Tonic Tea (page 170).

Pine Needles (Pinus spp.): The needles of most species of pine trees have both edible and medicinal properties. They are aromatic and have antibacterial and pain-relieving properties. Pine needles are high in vitamin C and are an effective expectorant for coughs. Pregnant women should avoid using the needles from ponderosa pine. Use pine needles in Pine Needle Cough Syrup (page 82).

Plantain (Plantago major): This common and easy-to-identify "weed" has strong anti-inflammatory and antimicrobial properties. Plantain is excellent for healing wounds and relieving itchiness from bites, stings and rashes. It is most often used externally as a poultice or in healing salves and balms. Use plantain in Four-Herb Wound Salve (page 62), Itchy Bite & Sting Balm (page 66), Eczema Relief Salve (page 97) and Diaper Rash Salve (page 181).

Red Clover (Trifolium pratense): This flower, which is common on lawns and grassy areas, is rich in vitamins and minerals. Red clover is a powerful blood and lymphatic cleanser, and it is good for respiratory ailments. It is also used to increase fertility and for menopausal issues. Pregnant women should avoid using red clover. Use red clover in Long Infusion Fertility Tea (page 169).

Red Raspberry Leaf (Rubus idaeus): The leaf of red raspberry is especially known as a tonic for women during pregnancy and postpartum. It is high in many vitamins and minerals and tones the uterus, possibly making labor easier. Red raspberry leaf is also beneficial for increasing fertility. Pregnant women should consult their doctor or midwife before taking red raspberry leaf, especially during the first trimester. Use red raspberry leaf in Long Infusion Fertility Tea (page 169), Pregnancy Tonic Tea (page 170) and Lactation Tea (page 173).

Rose (Rosa spp.): This popular garden flower has edible and medicinal uses. Both the flowers and the hips, which is the fruit that forms after the flowers, are beneficial. Rose petals are cooling and anti-inflammatory, and the flowers are often used in skin care recipes. Rose hips help to boost the immune system and are extremely high in vitamin C. Use rose in Super Immunity Infusion Tea (page 27), Vitamin C Tea (page 28), Rejuvenating Flower Bath Soak (page 136), Rose Petal & Rose Hip Face Serum (page 144) and Calendula & Rose Hip Immune-Boosting Glycerite (page 189).

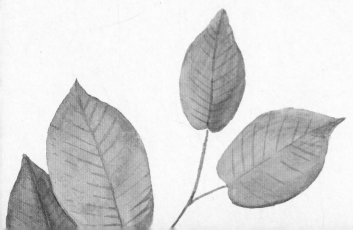

Rosemary (Rosmarinus officinalis): This common perennial garden herb is a brain tonic that helps to improve concentration and memory. It is also a mild and uplifting stimulant that eases headaches and depression, and it treats poor circulation and low blood pressure. Rosemary is anti-inflammatory and antioxidant as well as an effective pain reliever and immune system booster. It is also beneficial for the hair and scalp. Use rosemary in Fresh Kitchen Herb Oxymel (page 40), Herbal Hair Wash (page 159) and Rosemary & Thyme Flaky Scalp Treatment (page 163).

Sage (Salvia officinalis): This kitchen garden herb is a powerful immune booster and is helpful for fighting colds and flus. Sage is astringent and antiseptic, making it an effective remedy for sore throats and coughs. It is also beneficial for calming nerves and reducing stress. Lactating women should avoid using sage as it can dry up your supply. Use sage in Fermented Garlic, Ginger & Sage in Honey (page 35), Fresh Kitchen Herb Oxymel (page 40), Sage, Marshmallow & Ginger Sore Throat Tea (page 77), De-Stress Tea (page 127) and Herbal Hair Wash (page 159).

Sarsaparilla (Smilax ornata): The root of the sarsaparilla vine has traditionally been used in making old-fashioned root beer. It is high in anti-inflammatory saponins that gives it a bitter taste, and it is good for the digestive system. Sarsaparilla is also high in plant sterols and antioxidants. Use sarsaparilla in Sarsaparilla & Fennel Bitters (page 116).

Skullcap (Scutellaria lateriflora): This mint-family herb is an effective sedative and nerve tonic. It is antispasmodic and helps to relieve nervous tension, stress, anxiety and pain. Skullcap is also highly beneficial for reducing headache pain. Use skullcap in Headache Relief Tea (page 73).

Slippery Elm (Ulmus fulva): The inner bark of the slippery elm tree is highly mucilaginous and is excellent for reducing pain and inflammation. It is an effective digestive aid and is commonly used to treat sore throats and coughs. Due to unethical harvesting, slippery elm is considered to be an at-risk herb, so use sparingly and only buy from reputable sources. Marshmallow root makes a good sustainable alternative. Use slippery elm in Horehound Sore Throat Syrup (page 78).

Saint John's Wort (Hypericum perforatum): This plant with little yellow flowers grows wild almost everywhere as a "weed" that can easily be foraged. It is a highly effective nervine and sedative with strong antidepressant properties. Saint John's wort is also a powerful anti-inflammatory wound healer. Use Saint John's wort in the Saint John's Wort & Cayenne Warming Oil (page 53) and the Saint John's Wort Tincture for Lifting Low Spirits (page 131).

Sunflower (Helianthus annuus): This tall, bright and sunny flower is a common sight in summertime gardens, and surprisingly also has some medicinal benefits. It is high in antioxidants and is anti-inflammatory for the skin. Sunflower is often used in natural hair care products, adding shine and conditioning effects. Use sunflower in Sunflower, Violet Leaf & Mint Vinegar Hair Rinse (page 160).

Turmeric (Curcuma longa): This relative to ginger has a bright orange root that has powerful anti-inflammatory and pain-relieving properties, especially when paired with black pepper. Turmeric is also antibacterial, helps to boost the immune system and is a warming digestive aid. Use turmeric root in Immune-Boosting Vinegar Infusion (Hot or Not) (page 43), Turmeric & Black Pepper Tea for Chronic Inflammation (page 61) and Ginger & Turmeric Decoction & Honey Syrup (page 103).

Thyme (*Thymus vulgaris*): This common herb garden plant has powerful disinfectant properties that help to fight off infection. Thyme is a tonic herb with antifungal and immune-boosting benefits, and is excellent for treating sore throats, coughs and colds. Use thyme in Fermented Red Onion & Thyme in Honey (page 36), Fresh Kitchen Herb Oxymel (page 40), Immune-Boosting Vinegar Infusion (Hot or Not) (page 43), Basil, Thyme & Oregano Tea for Chronic Pain (page 58), Thyme, Peppermint & Honey Tea for Coughs (page 81), Herbal Hair Wash (page 159) and Rosemary & Thyme Flaky Scalp Treatment (page 163).

Uva Ursi (*Arctostaphylos uva-ursi*): Also known as bearberry or kinnikinnick, this low-growing evergreen shrub is highly beneficial for the urinary tract system. It is a powerful astringent and diuretic with antibacterial and antiseptic properties. Do not use uva ursi for more than a week at a time. Children ages 12 and under should not be given uva ursi. Use uva ursi in UTI Relief Tea (page 94).

Valerian Root (*Valeriana officinalis*): The root of the valerian flower is a highly effective nerve tonic treating stress, tension and insomnia. It is one of the best herbs for inducing sleep. Valerian is also a muscle relaxant, and it is beneficial for treating headaches and pain. For some people, valerian is stimulating; discontinue use as a sleep aid if you notice this effect. Use valerian root in Sleep Well Tea (page 124).

Violet Leaf (*Viola spp.*): This low-growing wild plant has small edible flowers that are usually purple, but sometimes white or yellow, and heart-shape leaves. Violet leaf is highly mucilaginous and emollient and is commonly used in skin care and hair care products. Use violet leaf in Dry Hands Balm (page 148), Sunflower, Violet Leaf & Mint Vinegar Hair Rinse (page 160) and Cradle Cap Oil (page 178).

White Willow Bark (*Salix alba*): The inner bark of the white willow tree has been used as medicine for many centuries, and it grows nearly everywhere. It contains the same compounds that are used to make aspirin, but it is much more gentle than over-the-counter aspirin. White willow bark is a powerful pain reliever, anti-inflammatory and blood thinner, and as a febrifuge it helps to reduce fevers. Use white willow bark in White Willow & Birch Bark Tea for Pain Relief (page 57).

Witch Hazel (*Hamamelis virginiana*): The bark and leaves of the witch hazel shrub are high in tannins and are very astringent. Witch hazel tea is used topically as a cooling and anti-inflammatory wound healer and as a general tonic for the skin. It is highly effective for treating hemorrhoids and when used in a soothing and healing postpartum bath. Do not take witch hazel internally. Use witch hazel in Witch Hazel & Blackberry Leaf Face Wash (page 156).

Yarrow (*Achillea millefolum*): This common wild plant has distinctive frilly leaves and flowers that are usually white, but they can also be pink, red, yellow or orange. Yarrow is a powerful wound healer and a poultice made from its leaves helps to clot the blood. It is antiseptic, anti-inflammatory, antispasmodic and diuretic. It is a cure-all plant and is an important one to know how to identify out in the wild. Those with ragweed allergies should avoid using yarrow. Pregnant women should avoid using yarrow internally. Use yarrow in Four-Herb Wound Salve (page 62), Fever-Reducing Tea (page 85) and UTI Relief Tea (page 94).

RESOURCES

BOOKS

These are the books on foraging, herbal medicine and natural skin care that I reach for most often and helped me to write this book.

Edible and Medicinal Plants in Wild (and Not So Wild) Places by "Wildman" Steve Brill

Medicinal Herbs: A Beginner's Guide by Rosemary Gladstar

Herbal Recipes for Vibrant Health by Rosemary Gladstar

The Herbal Medicine-Maker's Handbook by James Green

Making Plant Medicine by Richo Cech

101 Easy Homemade Products for Your Skin, Health, & Home by Jan Berry

WEBSITES

Grow Forage Cook Ferment—My blog! Follow me for foraging and wildcrafting tips, real-food recipes, fermenting and preserving recipes, gardening and permaculture ideas and herbalism inspiration. https://www.growforagecookferment.com/

The Nerdy Farm Wife—Jan Berry's blog has recipes for all-natural bath and beauty products, soap and herbal medicine. https://thenerdyfarmwife.com/

The Herbal Academy—A great place to take online courses about herbalism. They cover everything for beginners to more advanced students. https://theherbalacademy.com/

Chestnut School of Herbal Medicine—Another awesome place to take online herbal medicine and foraging courses. https://chestnutherbs.com/

SUPPLIES

Mountain Rose Herbs—This is where I buy almost all of my dried herbs and flowers that I don't forage myself. They are organic and very high quality. They also carry beeswax, butters, carrier oils, essential oils, small jars and tins, and most everything else you need for making DIY herbal products. https://www.mountainroseherbs.com/

Fillmore Container—They have an amazing selection of mason jars, as well as bottles and jars in all different shapes and sizes for storing your finished infusions. https://www.fillmorecontainer.com/

Excalibur Dehydrator—My favorite dehydrator, this is what I make most of my infused oils in because they have low temperature settings and I can fit many jars in at one time. https://www.excaliburdehydrator.com/

Azure Standard—This free-to-join food buying club is the best place to buy high-quality and organic products in bulk, such as raw honey, coconut and olive oils and raw apple cider vinegar. https://www.azurestandard.com/

HERBAL PRODUCTS

Coco's Herbals Etsy Shop—This is my Etsy shop where I sell handmade salves, balms and lotion bars, including some that are recipes in this book. https://www.etsy.com/shop/CocosHerbals

ACKNOWLEDGMENTS

First, a huge thank you to the readers of my blog, Grow Forage Cook Ferment. You are all amazing, and this book wouldn't be here without your continuing support!

Big thanks to Will Kiester and everyone at Page Street Publishing for taking on this little herbalism book. A special shout-out to my editor, Sarah Monroe, for being so patient and guiding me along every step of the way.

Thank you so much to Jan Berry for suggesting me to Page Street and for answering all of my questions in a kind and thoughtful way throughout the whole process. You are an inspiration!

Special thanks to my fellow blogging ladies: Teri, Kathie, Kris, Devon, Susan, Isis, Quinn, Amy S., Janet, Angi, Jess, Chris, Connie, Rachel, Shelle, Tanya, Amy F., Amanda, Ann, Abigail, Meredith, Tessa, Megan, Dawn and Amy D. You are super awesome. Thank you for all of your love and support through thick and thin!

Thanks to Jennifer Anne Nelson for your beautiful herb and flower drawings; they made this book extra special! To see more of Jen's artwork, visit her website here: https://www.itsjenniferanne.com/

And thanks to The Wondersmith for providing me with your amazing handmade ceramic mug for the Roasted Chicory Root Chai photo! To see more of The Wondersmith's work, visit their website here: https://www.thewondersmith.com/

Thank you to my sister, Katy, for keeping me grounded, listening to me with an open mind, providing solid advice and making me laugh along the way. You are an amazing sister and friend!

Much love to my mom Robin for always believing in me no matter what and thinking that I'm the best at what I do. I wouldn't be who I am without you. And to my dad who is no longer on this planet but I know would be proud of the person I have become.

Thanks and love to my husband Joel, who helped me at every step of the way to make this book happen. You are an amazing partner and father, and I literally couldn't have done it without you! And to my baby boy Sawyer, this book is for you, so that you can live a life surrounded in natural elements whenever possible. I will teach you the way of the plants.

And last but not least, to Mother Earth who provides us with everything that we need to heal, we just need to pay attention to what she is saying.

ABOUT THE AUTHOR

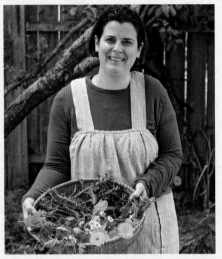

Colleen Codekas lives with her husband Joel and their son Sawyer in the beautiful Rogue Valley of southern Oregon, where they have created a mini permaculture paradise. Due to her desire to live in the most natural way possible, she began studying herbs and herbal medicine nearly 20 years ago. Living and working in Yosemite National Park for 10 years, many of those spent in the high elevation paradise of Tuolumne Meadows, solidified a yearning for being surrounded by nature on a daily basis. Learning to correctly identify wild plants, particularly those that were edible and medicinal, became a new hobby while living in the wilderness, and has carried over into her more "traditional" life now. In recent years, Colleen has completed several herbalism courses through the Herbal Academy and continues to teach people what she knows through her blog Grow Forage Cook Ferment. When she isn't busy writing for her blog or making things for her Etsy shop, Coco's Herbals, she likes to go foraging for wild, edible and medicinal plants and mushrooms. She also enjoys hiking, cooking delicious food, drinking wine, making mead, growing a ridiculous amount of herbs and flowers and making all kinds of herbal goodness in jars.

INDEX

Healing Herbal Infusions